show
up

Tammy Hembrow is an entrepreneur and one of Australia's most successful creators, with over 20 million followers. As the founder of fitness platform Tammy Fit and luxury athleisure label Saski, Tammy's mission is to motivate and inspire people to feel their best. Tammy has been listed in *Business News Australia*'s 40 under 40, won Young Entrepreneur of the Year Australia in her category for *Business News Australia*, and been voted *Cosmopolitan* magazine's Social Media Star of the Year, Fitness & Travel. She is mum to Wolf, Saskia and Posy.

 @tammyhembrow

show up

up

Mindset, motivation and creating your dream life

Tammy Hembrow

EBURY
PRESS

EBURY PRESS

UK | USA | Canada | Ireland | Australia
India | New Zealand | South Africa | China

Ebury Press is part of the Penguin Random House group of companies
whose addresses can be found at global.penguinrandomhouse.com.

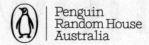

First published by Ebury Press 2024

Cover photography by Carlene Raschke
Cover design by Adam Laszczuk © Penguin Random House Australia Pty Ltd
Typeset in 12.5/16 pt Bembo by Midland Typesetters, Australia

Printed and bound in Australia by Griffin Press, an accredited
ISO AS/NZS 14001 Environmental Management Systems printer

 A catalogue record for this
book is available from the
National Library of Australia

ISBN 978 1 76134 383 4

penguin.com.au

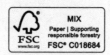

*We at Penguin Random House Australia acknowledge that Aboriginal and Torres Strait Islander
peoples are the Traditional Custodians and the first storytellers of the lands on which we live and work.
We honour Aboriginal and Torres Strait Islander peoples' continuous connection to Country, waters,
skies and communities. We celebrate Aboriginal and Torres Strait Islander stories, traditions and living
cultures; and we pay our respects to Elders past and present.*

To everyone showing up even when they don't feel like it – when they're busy, when they're feeling unmotivated or in a slump. Keep going. Keep showing up. That's when it counts the most. ♡

CONTENTS

People think
they know you
from the outside,
but it's what
drives you from
the inside that
counts.

PROLOGUE

If you asked me to pinpoint where my journey began, I could tell you *exactly*. Picture me, twelve years old, wild blonde hair tumbling around my head, sitting on a comfy leather lounge and surrounded by books as far as the eye can see. Technically, this is my home. But it feels as far from home as I could ever have imagined.

The day before, I had waved goodbye to my ramshackle childhood house in Australia, to my free-spirited, lovable father, and to my tiny primary school of just eighty kids. I'd hopped on a plane and flown through the night to come and live with my mum, step-dad and two sisters in Singapore – a city taller than it was wide, with skyscrapers that kissed the sky. Unlike my father who'd given up his fledgling acting career to raise three girls alone in the Queensland rainforest, my step-dad was a hugely successful international businessman. The books surrounding me were his personal library, rows upon rows of them, all willing me to become their new friend.

I was fascinated. I mean, seriously, who has an actual library in their own house? I remember walking along the shelves, touching the spines, reading the titles. *The Success Principles* by Jack Canfield, *Think and Grow Rich* by Napoleon Hill, *Rich Dad*

Poor Dad by Robert Kiyosaki – every single book a declaration of personal empowerment and self-driven success.

I don't know where my sisters were – this house was so big, I kept losing everyone. But I was alone and bored and *very* curious. So I picked up a book, made myself comfy and started reading. Little did I know, I was on the brink of a whole new adventure. Coming to Singapore had been the start of my journey, but reading these books and learning how my step-dad had built his wealth opened my mind in ways I hadn't known were possible. As soon as I finished the first book, I started reading another, then another, then another.

*

Several years later, my brain expanded from all the reading, my heart expanded from all the family time and my horizons expanded from all the travel we'd done, it was time for me to head back to Australia. Taking one last look around my step-dad's library, I recalled that little girl who'd picked up her first book all those years ago and realised just how much I had changed. It wasn't simply that life had been different in Singapore; *I* had become different in Singapore. Reading those books had ignited something within me. I wanted to create a similar life for myself; to use my mind, my drive and my ambition to have an impact on the world. I didn't know what yet, or how, but I did know one thing: that whatever it was, I'd do it my way, as my own boss.

I'd begun to dream big, believing I could create something amazing. I knew it was possible. When people ask about my success, I always say it boils down to mindset. My teenage years in Singapore – reading those books, travelling the world and watching my step-dad's success – had forged a strength in me. Without even realising it, I had begun to back myself. Now all I needed was an idea and motivation . . . and to show up.

INTRODUCTION

Welcome to *Show Up*! I'm excited and, if I'm being honest, maybe a touch nervous, to open myself up and share my experiences with you in these pages. I don't pretend to have all the answers. I've experienced some incredible success – thanks to plenty of hard work, determination and a positive mindset – but I've also had my fair share of ups and downs.

If your journey is anything like mine, it will be tough at times, but uplifting too. The secret, I've found, is that no matter what's going on around you, if you make the commitment to show up for yourself day every single day, no matter how you're feeling, then you have every chance to create the life of your dreams.

People see my 20 million Instagram followers and TikTok reels of my three smiling kids, two successful businesses and close friendship with my sisters and believe I'm living the ultimate fantasy – a dream that's impossible for them to achieve. But the truth is, I'm just a regular Aussie girl at heart. I grew up in sub-tropical Queensland, in the Currumbin Valley, in a house with no bedroom walls and an outside bath. Barefoot and free-spirited, I attended the tiny, local primary school with a handful of other kids. Back then, no-one, least of all me, would have dreamt I'd be living the life I live now. Simply through self-belief and a lot of effort, I have managed to create a life that I adore. And you can too.

This book will show you the real story behind my social media success – the mistakes, the wins and the steps I took to create it. You'll read about the paths I've travelled and some of the people I've met along the way – the good, the bad and the ugly. Whether you're here to learn about my fitness tips, the secrets to my business success, or what relationships mean to me, I'll cover it all. Alongside my stories, I'll share some of the practical tips and strategies that have worked for me. Perhaps some will help you build your own sparkling future – whatever that looks like for you.

Of all the things I stand for, the most important is knowing who you are, believing in yourself, and backing yourself with intention and hard work. You are the *only you* in the universe, so what you imagine for your ideal life will be different from mine or my sisters' or anyone else's out there. I'm not here to show you how to live like Tammy Hembrow, but hopefully, by hearing my story, you'll be inspired to create your own best life.

This is *not* a book about aiming for perfection or meeting other people's expectations of you. It's a book about fulfilling your potential in the areas that truly matter, while retaining your authentic self as you set your own standards for success. All of it begins with one basic idea, the one I learnt in Singapore and live by every day: to show up – for yourself, for your dreams and for those you care about.

For me, as a lot of you will know, showing up means starting my day early. With three kids and two businesses to run, I know I have to get up with the sun. But do I leap out of bed grinning every morning? No, of course not! Sometimes yes, but often no. I can think of a million excuses to stay in bed at 5 a.m – sometimes I just lie there for a sec and go, *really?*

But I've learnt that if you focus on your priority, getting up and going for it is pretty easy. Once you turn your mind to your 'why', it doesn't take long to get excited about the day ahead. And so, I get up. I show up. I remind myself how good I will feel

The amount of times in my life I've been told that my goals or what I want is 'unrealistic' . . . Never did and never will listen. Go create whatever reality you want, baby!

after I work out, how much more time I will have in the day by starting early, and how much 'habit making' and 'habit keeping' drives my success.

My wins, big and small, are the result of keeping a strong body and a strong mind. If there's one thing I absolutely know about backing yourself and being the best version of you, it's that mindset is *everything*. Your thoughts create who you are: they drive your actions, which dictate your mood, which affects how you interact with others and, ultimately, what you achieve. For me, it's easy to see how your 'thoughts become things'. I am a fan of manifesting because that's where big dreams begin. And when you dream, plan and execute – that's how life gets made. Starting your day with your dreams front and centre, you realise you can achieve almost *anything*. If you simply get up, show up, and keep putting one foot in front of the other, over time you'll find that you – and your life – will change.

But it's not easy! I am still working at creating a life that's *balanced*. A lot of my early success was down to me putting a hundred per cent of my focus into my businesses, sometimes at the expense of my family, my friends and my health. I've learnt that maintaining a balanced life is hard, but so, so worth it. It is not something you can just 'set and forget'. Life is always changing and so are your priorities. Sometimes this means putting all your effort into a particular area to grow it while allowing another area to coast.

In this book I cover eight key areas of life:
- work
- relationships
- movement
- nourishment
- parenting
- challenges
- development
- celebration.

INTRODUCTION

Achieving balance isn't about perfection, it's about doing what you need to do for *you* on any given day. It's about responding *in the moment* and making the most of every opportunity. 'Having it all' means you must juggle your priorities and compromise. In order to do that well, you need to know what matters to *you* and focus on that. So my greatest piece of advice is this: listen to that voice inside. Let your inner guide dictate where you put your attention and who you give it to.

I hope my words inspire you to find your own path and figure out what will help you live your best life. Whatever dreams you may have, if you want them enough, and you show up and back yourself, you can create the life you want. It's completely up to you.

WORK

I've always liked that saying, 'If you love what you do, you'll never work a day in your life.' These days, I love how I earn my living, but like most people, there was a time when I had a job I absolutely hated and didn't have a clue what I wanted to do. When I was very young, I wanted to be an actress. I'm not really sure why, I just always wanted something 'big' for myself; something larger than life. Given my dad was an actor, maybe it came from him, but mostly I think it came from the childhood he encouraged us to lead.

The Currumbin Valley is a lush, tropical oasis near the Gold Coast, yet, as rich as the landscape was, our little family was anything but. The part of the rainforest where we lived had a small population but it was such a close-knit, happy community. My parents had divorced early on, so my sisters and I lived with my dad on a farm. It sounds funny to say, but we didn't even have a proper house. We lived in an old wedding reception venue – a small hall with walls made out of tables turned on their sides and doors made of tacked-up blankets. We had to fill the outdoor bathtub with hot water from a kettle. Dad called it an 'adventure' and I suppose it was, in a way.

I've always told myself it's possible to have it all. To be a full-time mum as well as a successful, hands-on business owner. To strive for success and the finer things, while staying grounded and grateful for the smallest blessings in life.

Dad is creative and eccentric, loud and larger than life, and my childhood in the Currumbin Valley involved a lot of outdoor play and inventing games. When my dad was younger, he acted in both the theatre and on TV, and was somewhat famous in Australia. He's also a musician and can play almost any instrument he picks up. There was never a dull moment in our household. We might have lived in an old hall and rarely watched TV, but it was the best childhood *ever*. Ours was a true home, filled with music, imagination and fun. I'll always be thankful to my dad for allowing my wild, dreamy side to flourish as a barefoot flower child.

By the time I turned twelve, however, I was ready for something more. My two older sisters had moved to Singapore months earlier to live with my mum and step-dad, while I was finishing primary school. Once they gave it the all-clear, I made the decision to move there too. On the verge of becoming a teen, it was time for me to spread my wings and see what else the world had to offer. Plus – as much as I didn't like to admit it then – a girl needs her mum and sisters.

Though my parents didn't get along, it wasn't a matter of choosing one over the other, it was simply an opportunity to try something new and see how it went for a while. I knew Dad would miss us, but he was always really supportive of us chasing our dreams. I was so nervous. I was about to begin high school, so the idea of packing up and starting somewhere new was a massive deal, especially as I am naturally a shy person. But when it all came down to it, I missed my sisters and my mum, so I pushed myself out of my comfort zone and decided to give it a go.

It was literally a life-changing decision.

Singaporean life was *the polar opposite* of life back home, especially when I discovered that library and all those books. The minute I opened my first one, I felt like I was unlocking the secrets to a whole new universe. I didn't know what or how or when, but I knew without a doubt that my entire world had shifted.

Do what you love and it won't be work, it'll be your passion.

FIND YOUR
PASSION

For most people, it's not easy figuring out what to do with your life, let alone how to turn your passion into a lifestyle. Believe it or not, I was one of those people. For a long time, I had absolutely no idea what I wanted to do, only that I wanted to make it big! The best way to find your direction is to give things a go.

Sometimes I think how different my life might have been if I hadn't gone to Singapore. You *do* need to get out of your comfort zone sometimes. Sitting around and overthinking things will often make a situation worse, while getting up and trying something new will bring a shift. Before I discovered my passion, I tried plenty of things that didn't work out, including going to university and a job I really hated.

*

Back in Australia, I enrolled in a business degree. I didn't do it because I saw it as my career pathway, I just couldn't face taking on a nine-to-five job. I figured that since the degree had the word 'business' in it, it might give me a chance of following in my step-dad's entrepreneurial footsteps.

I soon realised that this particular university course wasn't the kind of business dream I had in mind *at all* and, despite getting

13

good grades, subjects like Economics 101 weren't doing it for me. Truthfully? I hated it and, like for so many other high-school leavers, the years after I left were pretty crappy. There's so much pressure, making that big decision about what to do with the rest of your life, and most of us have *no* idea. Even though the person probably means well, when I hear people asking teenagers, 'What are you planning to do after school?', I just want to step in and protect them.

How is anyone at that age supposed to just 'know'? That pressure was something I didn't cope with well at all and having seen what people in Singapore were capable of made me feel, in a way, even more useless, indecisive and inadequate. At that point, I spiralled down in a pretty bad way. I was partying hard and smoking weed, which only made me sadder. My energy and motivation to do anything vanished. I became lost and depressed and didn't know how to climb out of the hole I found myself in.

Then someone suggested meditation and yoga. Lucky for me, I've always been open to trying new things. *Get out of your comfort zone, Tammy*, I thought. I was in a pretty low state, so I figured anything was worth a shot. How hard could it be? I opened a meditation app, thinking I'd be told to chill and take some deep breaths. Little did I know, I was about to have my mind *blown*.

Guided into a deeply relaxed state, I became hyper-aware of every molecule in my body. My imagination kicked into action. With the deep breathing acting like a drug, I felt like I was being scanned energetically and healing with each inhale/exhale. In that moment, I learnt the meaning of being 'truly present'. At the same time it felt like I was having an out-of-body experience. When it was over, I felt completely transformed.

Meditation led to yoga, where I began training as an instructor. From there, the world of weight training and fitness opened up. Moving my body each day began to recalibrate my mind. It was like a light had been switched on, illuminating what had been a dark place. It was as if the exercise and mind-work had unlocked the universe. Suddenly, and with complete clarity, I knew exactly what I wanted to do with my life. I *knew* what my passion was.

Give it a go

Have you ever tried something new and thoroughly enjoyed it? Maybe there's something you used to love doing that you haven't done for a while. Either way, could you make more time for it . . . could it even become your passion? Your career?

Here are a few ideas to prompt you. Circle the ones that appeal and maybe add in a few more. Come back and revisit this list often, continuing to try new things until something clicks. Doing what you love is always a good idea and, who knows, it may just lead to you getting paid for it. It did for me.

Things to try:

Organising social events

Going to new places

Working out

Meditating

Planning an adventure

Creating imaginary worlds

Taking up music

Trying a new hobby

Other: ....

Your inner journey reflects your
outer one. ✿ I love working out
& working on my physical form,
it's a kind of therapy for me. But
your mind is something even
more important to work on . . .
I challenge you to start doing
5–10 minutes of mindfulness in
the morning or evening. See how
it makes you feel, see how your
life evolves & changes: your
sense of peace, your mood, your
mindset, and in turn, your actions
& your life.

If someone else
can do it, why
not you?

DREAM BIG

It's funny how our mind plays tricks on us. We find ourselves saying we *can't* do something for so many reasons, which often are simply not true. One thing I started asking myself in my step-dad's library is, *If these people I'm reading about can do this, why **not** me?* Meanwhile, my inner critic was shouting back, *Because you're young, you're a woman, you don't have the money, the connections, the experience!* But the more I read, the stronger my self-belief became.

As it turned out, I started Tammy Fit as a young woman with no money and no connections. I made my own opportunities, took action, and eventually found success. While those negative thoughts may have had some basis in reality, I chose not to let them take hold and dictate my actions. Instead, I chose to believe I could overcome those so-called obstacles and forge new paths. As I say, mindset is everything.

I often hear people moan that they 'don't have the capacity', or that they're 'too tired, busy or overwhelmed' or that 'it's not the right time'. If this thing is in your heart, then now is *always* the right time to pursue it. Because if not now, when? And if not you . . . who?

*

Once I'd figured out what my passion was, it was pretty easy to see how I could make it into a career. By then, I was nearing the end of my business degree and had finally found a subject I enjoyed: entrepreneurship. Logically, that should have driven me to stay on and finish my final few subjects and earn my degree, but it had the opposite effect – I felt I'd learnt everything I needed to know. So, I walked straight out the door and didn't come back. I didn't care that I was so close to graduating, because why wait to start my big dream? Seriously, *why even wait a single day*? I was ready to kick some goals.

With every ounce of my being, I was certain of three things:

1. Mental/physical health and fitness was my passion.
2. What I'd learnt in my step-dad's library and studying entrepreneurship was all the knowledge I needed.
3. All I had to do now was to get out there and back myself and this would happen.

Don't ask me why I was certain of that last one, I just was. I'd known ever since I'd been that dreamy kid running around the forest. I'd known as a teenager in a strange new world, sitting down and reading a heap of self-development and business books. I'd always known these things were possible and I knew it would happen for me. I'd read thousands of stories about it and seen others' success play out. Why *not* me?

Look, I'm aware that most people would think that dropping out of uni at the age of nineteen and deciding to be an entrepreneur isn't exactly a well-timed and well-considered plan. But for me, I knew it was. How?

I believe that the time is right when your passion is high. Motivation and mindset are everything – you need *all of it* to take that first, most important step. Stepping off the edge takes courage and the best time to do it is when you've decided, *This is what I want*. That moment is your commitment. The time your dream begins is the minute you make the decision. It's like turning the car key and releasing the handbrake. Once you're on the journey, the fastest way to get to your destination is to keep going.

So keep going. Let that early momentum pitch you forward and use it to stay ahead.

Your turn to shine

Achieving your dreams starts with imagining them, then believing that they're possible. You have to believe this with all your conviction. When you want something to happen and believe that something *will* happen, you take active, practical steps to make it so: you turn on a light switch to get rid of the dark, you make a quick snack to beat hunger, or you call a friend to boost your mood. First you dream, then you act, and so it shall be. Let's practise.

First, answer these questions:

1. What's a dream you'd love to make happen?

....

....

....

2. Who do you know who's achieved this, either in your life or out in the world?

....

....

....

Now, close your eyes and imagine how you would feel having achieved that dream. Spend a couple of minutes visualising this in as much detail as possible: what you're wearing, what smells are in the air, what sort of space you're in and who you're with. Make your vision as real and as detailed as possible, then respond to these questions, answering as if your dream has come true and you are experiencing it in the present.

I am feeling ....

....

....

Because ....

....

....

My life is now so ....

....

....

I started a business degree majoring in marketing . . . I had one month left, then dropped out. The only class I liked was entrepreneurship – it was just so practical and spot-on. I'm not saying people should not go to uni or not finish uni, it's just that with me, it wasn't something I wanted or needed to get where I wanted to be.

Create your own
reality, baby!

PROVE 'EM WRONG

It's one thing to find your passion, have big dreams and decide to do something with them, but sadly, not everyone is going to be on board with your decisions. Many who love you are also protective of you, so they'll often be cautious and urge you to play it safe.

Perhaps, like me, you've heard this sort of thing: 'No, no – you should finish your degree first' or 'Just do that part-time job and save for a rainy day' or 'First things first, experience and references are what matters'. Safe, safe, safe. Meanwhile all that burning ambition is burning *out* and before you know it, you're stuck in the 'existing instead of living' rut that is so common.

If you are happy with your life, that's great! But if you're not . . . if you're making decisions to please everyone else and satisfy their expectations, then it's time for a shake-up. You only get one life and, in the end, what you do with it should be up to you. It's fine, when we're kids, to rely on our parents and teachers to guide us. But one of the benefits of adulting is taking control of your own life. It's time to take charge of your destiny.

*

Any time someone told me no, it just made me push that much harder. Don't ever let anyone or anything stop you. More importantly, don't let your own THOUGHTS stop you. Behind every successful person I know is the BELIEF they can and will succeed. So make sure you are backing yourself.

I found myself in exactly this position when I decided I was done with uni and would instead follow my passion. Luckily, I managed to convince my family I was making the right decision.

But then life decided to throw a curve ball: I discovered that I was pregnant. Suddenly I was surrounded by people telling me that my dreams were *impossible*.

Was I shocked? Yes. Did it in any way stop me from pursuing my dreams? Absolutely not. As far as I was concerned, *nothing* had changed. I knew that meditation, yoga, health and fitness had potentially saved my life, so I sure as hell wasn't about to stop doing them now. In fact, it made me *more* determined than ever to spread the word about how important they are. Being pregnant would just have to be a part of that journey. In fact, why not make it a *key* part of the journey?

As you might expect, not everyone agreed with my approach. 'What do you mean you want to start your own business? You're nineteen years old and you're having a baby!' said one. Others said I'd ruined my life, that my body would never be the same (so good luck being some kind of fitness guru!), and what would I know about becoming a successful businesswoman anyway. Another said, 'A teenage mum with *nothing* to show for herself has *no chance* of becoming an entrepreneur.'

People thought it was far more logical – in other words, safe, safe, safe – to do some crappy job instead. To look after the baby with my boyfriend as best I could. But what kind of life and future would that give me? I was determined to do more. To *be* more.

Of course those warnings rattled me. Of course it was a lot to deal with. But the second I started feeling defeated, I rallied. If anything, their words made me *more* determined to prove them wrong! I'm stubborn like that. When people tell me I can't do something, it encourages me to go harder. I've never really allowed myself to slip into the mindset of believing something is 'too hard' or 'unrealistic' and I hate it when people use that term to describe my life. I believe we create our own reality – what's so unrealistic about that?

With my mindset firmly in place, I ignored them. I set myself the firm intention of becoming a successful businesswoman *and* a young mum. I had my dreams and goals and was determined to prove the naysayers wrong. Just because plans change, doesn't mean your dreams have to as well.

Cultivate self-belief

There are lots of great things you can do to boost your self-belief, such as listing ten things you like about yourself, or reading old birthday cards, but here's something I've found to be incredibly powerful. I call it the Top Ten Success List and it's so effective, I still use it whenever I need a confidence boost.

It's pretty straightforward – list ten things you've achieved in life. Funnily enough, writing this list can be tough because most of us work so hard to be humble. But now is not the time for humility. List ten things you've accomplished. Go!

1. ....

2. ....

3. ....

4. ....

5. ....

6. ....

7. ....

8. ....

9. ....

10. ....

Begin with what you have, the rest you'll figure out along the way.

WHAT YOU
CAN CONTROL

You've decided to take charge of your life. Good for you! And so you find yourself in the driver's seat of life's metaphorical car when it occurs to you, *I don't exactly know where I'm going . . .* Is it time to freak out? I don't think so. Stop for a minute and ask yourself – honestly, does anyone *really* know where they're going? As you saw with my first pregnancy, life has a habit of throwing curve balls, some of which we have zero control over.

The only thing we can really influence is our attitude – how we respond to things. Which is why I love my step-dad's advice to never complain. 'Listen,' he said, 'if there's something you don't like that you can change, then change it, don't complain about it. And if you can't change it, then what's the point in complaining about it?'

Don't focus on what you *can't* control. Instead, change the situation if you can and your attitude if you can't; the glass isn't half-empty, it's half-full. If we only focused on the bad stuff, none of us would ever get out of bed. Where you put your focus is your choice, so focus on what you have and what you can control, not what you can't.

*

That was my attitude starting out, anyway. My initial goal was simple: share all the things I loved about exercising, food and mindfulness with the world. Surely it couldn't be that hard?

Surprisingly, it wasn't. My studies had taught me that you can start with nothing. Since I wasn't far off nothing, I really loved the idea that you can begin with what you have and figure out the rest along the way. Besides, I did have one thing: an Instagram account.

Although it was early days, it was already a great platform for reaching people. At that point, I had no idea just how many people I'd end up connecting with – influencers weren't a thing back then – but I had fun using it, and my followers were growing, so I kept posting. Lucky for me, I got in on the ground floor. I'd started posting because I liked fashion, taking photos and having fun with it, and somehow it had gained me an audience. I remember thinking when I reached 15,000 followers that it was a *huge* amount. Though other celebrities had way higher numbers, very few seemed to be capitalising on it. I could see so much potential and I found that super exciting.

However, my real job wasn't. Pregnant and barely making ends meet, I was working in a clothing store, trying to save as much as possible to finance my business. My only relief was going to the gym. I worked out five days a week and posted about it constantly – the highlight of my days.

I copped my fair share of criticism, with a lot of people saying I was being irresponsible exercising while pregnant. But I took my health more seriously than anyone and had regular check-ups with my doctor throughout my pregnancy. Based on my health and fitness levels, he was perfectly happy for me to continue with the exercise I'd been doing, which my body was used to.

For all the haters, I had twice as many supporters. Most people loved that I was young and pregnant and filled with positivity, motivation and aspirations. I showed that being pregnant

Life is a balancing act. If you lean too far one way, you'll fall. That's okay. Just make sure you get back up & try again. 🌅 Most of my life has been trying to balance being a mum, running my businesses & everything in between.

doesn't equate to an ending, rather, the beginning of a new way forward. In my experience, people seem to forget that pregnant women are still people – filled with ambition, energy, ideas and determination. If anything, I think pregnancy amps up those qualities up in me, and I've heard many other pregnant women say the same.

I was filled with passion and purpose and I was determined to have it all: a successful business, a baby, an amazing life – everything I wanted. My life wasn't 'over', it was simply my new (and improved) normal and I wanted to inspire other women to believe the same. You can still have a full life when you're pregnant. You can still have a full life with young children.

The more I posted, the more I could see the belief blossoming in others which further inspired my ideas and creativity. My gym posts got so many likes and comments, I decided to produce a workout program for my followers . . . but how was I going to create it when I was working elsewhere, growing a baby and trying to keep up my own health and fitness? Increasingly, it seemed like I would have to build my business full-time. But that would take more than moving out of a comfort zone – it would require an enormous leap of faith.

Change your perspective

Being honest with yourself, do you look at situations in your life as *glass half-full* or *glass half-empty*? Fill in this table and try to see both sides of the coin. Which column comes more easily to you? Can you catch yourself in the future and replace your negative thinking with a more positive way of looking things?

Situation	Glass half-empty	Glass half-full
It's raining.	I can't take the dog for our morning walk.	I can lie in bed reading without feeling guilty.

You'll only learn how to swim by letting go of the edge.

PROS AND CONS – WHEN IS THE TIME 'RIGHT'?

Relinquishing job security is like letting go of the edge of the pool when you're learning to swim. It can be seriously hard to give up a wage, because for all your dreaming about following your passion, giving up a salary to pursue it means this crazy idea just got real. It's one of the hardest moments in backing yourself because you literally *are* backing yourself – financially.

Ultimately, this affects how you can spend your leisure time, whether you can afford a holiday, or a house, or any other dreams you may have. If you forgo actual income, how does the rest of your life work? I'm saying this because no matter how lofty your dreams, you need one foot in inspiration-motivation land and one foot in pay-the-bills-reality land. Too much in either direction = unhappy. Getting the balance just right = amazing life. So how do you know when to let go?

*

Before I went full-time into creating Tammy Fit, my jobs had sucked. Before retail I'd worked as a telemarketer, making phone call after phone call, trying to sell solar panels. People had hung up on me all the time and I'd often cried after my shifts.

37

Meanwhile, I kept posting my life, fashion and gym sessions, growing this great following, and I had an idea for the perfect product. To make it happen, I needed to give it my full attention, yet my depressing day job was paying the bills. So how did I decide when the perfect time was to let go of the edge of that pool? I checked in with my internal barometer.

I'm a pretty positive person, but working those crummy jobs, I could feel myself getting depressed. Fitness had saved me once before and though I used it daily now, the dark edges were creeping back in. I knew if they got too close, I'd have to move quickly to stay afloat. I looked hard at my current situation, assessed it regularly and made a list. In one column were the 'reasons to stay' and in the other 'the reasons to go'.

Why stay?

- As shitty as this job is, it can help bring my dream to fruition.
- Every day I save a little more, which will help finance my dream.
- Fixed hours mean I can time-block my days to include working on my side hustle.
- I'm developing useful skills which I can use in my future business.
- I have access to networking, materials and other resources that I can't reach on my own.

Why go?

- It's the worst feeling ever, doing something you dread each day.
- I'm so tired, I don't have any energy to start building my future dream.
- This job is undermining my confidence and self-belief.
- I hardly make enough to pay the bills, let alone save for my dream.

In the end, it comes down to timing and how much you can personally handle. Being me, I got out as soon as I had the bare minimum for what I needed – in my case, a whole $400.

Balancing mum-life/work-life can be so incredibly hard sometimes. But it is beyond rewarding. Feeling so motivated at the moment & as always, trusting the process.

That's what I needed to produce the PDFs I was planning to make. Once I had that saved, I could launch my business. My baby hadn't arrived yet, so I had only myself to support and the sooner I built my dream, the better.

The timing was ideal. I hadn't overstayed to the point that the job had dragged me down, yet I had managed to build a little nest egg. But everyone has different needs and pain points. Before you make any big changes, sit down and think about what makes you happy and what might bring you unstuck. If leaving your job will make you so anxious that you can't focus on building your dream, maybe you need to keep earning a salary for a while longer as you build your business on the side.

One thing is certain, if starting your own business is your goal, it requires a huge amount of time and energy to get it off the ground. No doubt, you'll be working harder than you ever have on anything in your life, but the very big upside is that you'll be working on something you love and something wholly for you which you have full control over. Most likely, that will make you happier. Completely worth it, if you ask me.

What are you procrastinating about?

Here are five ways to take action and make it happen:

- ✓ Define your end goal and focus your attention on reaching it, not on the obstacles along the way. Set aside time each day to visualise having achieved it, in as much detail as possible.

- ✓ Make an action plan that's broken down into achievable small steps. Write them down or put reminders in your phone.

- ✓ Do something towards it every day, no matter how small. For example, if it's a trip you're planning, then make a shortlist of places to go and start comparing prices.

✓ Make a non-negotiable savings plan. If you're putting away $50 a week, transfer it to an account you can't easily access.

✓ Have fun along the way. Planning and achieving should be enjoyable! The more you think of life as one big game, the less stressful it is.

Your points of
difference make
you uniquely
you.

PERSPECTIVE IS EVERYTHING

It's funny looking back on ourselves as kids. Remember that boy who loved to draw horses and play handball every lunchtime; the girl who braided her hair and could run faster than anyone else; the loud one; the quiet one; the one who made you laugh? What were *you* like as a kid? Maybe you were naturally shy like me, but have since learnt to push yourself. Or maybe you were crazy-loud and grew into a quieter adult.

Whoever you were then, and whoever you are now, we all have in-built tendencies. You may have changed in subtle ways, but those tendencies will always be there – they are your foundation stone. I've always thought that it's important to remember the kid you once were. You're as unique now as you ever were, only, as adults, most of us try to fit into the grown-up world way too much. There's a whole lot of 'you should be this' going on: responsible, respectable, conforming. But you know something? You're still that kid. *You're still unique.*

Your points of difference make you uniquely you. That's what makes you special. There's no-one in the world like you – and all the weird, out-there stuff that maybe you've toned down or hidden away over the years is actually awesome. They're your super powers. Embrace them, use them, make them yours.

Perspective is everything. Your perspective and how you view things is so, so important. You can choose to view things one way or another. For example, you can say, 'I'm helpless, life hates me, I'm so unlucky!' Or you can say, 'I'm growing, I'm learning, I'm healing.' Every experience is a learning experience. You're growing as a person. Be kind enough to yourself to look at it that way instead.

It's worked for me. And my sisters. And most people I know who seem to have 'made something' of themselves. Part of that is standing out from the crowd, and the easiest way to do that is to be authentically you. When I began Tammy Fit, I was a shy, young, pregnant woman sharing my passion for the gym, health and fitness on Instagram – not exactly what you'd call 'normal'. But people loved it. They loved that I was working out with a baby bump and a huge grin I couldn't wipe off my face. They even loved my over-large teeth, which for most of my childhood, I hated. Thanks to people embracing the real me, I have come to appreciate myself a whole lot more – yes, even my toothy smile!

People love it when others show their innermost self and don't hide behind some fake mask of perfection. I'm not saying you can't look gorgeous, I'm talking about letting your inner light shine through. Think about your best friends – what do you love about them most? I bet it's their funny, crazy, imperfect and loveable ways.

So don't be afraid to be the *real* you. For every person who doesn't like you for it, there'll be ten who do. And the most important person on that list is you. Not wasting energy pretending to be someone you're not is an amazing gift of freedom. Imagine how much more you'll be able to do with your life when all that worry is redirected to making your dreams come true. All you have to do is be you.

*

I remember being worried about this when I left my boring-but-safe telemarketing job and started this entrepreneur gig for real. I mean, was anyone going to take me seriously?

Turns out I didn't have anything to worry about. People loved my workouts. My pregnancy and youth gave me a point of difference. Being publicly very pregnant and vulnerable to criticism while working out with my belly on show was a strength, not a weakness; an opportunity, not an obstacle. It meant I could encourage women while being honest about where I was at. And it worked. It resonated with people. I always say it came down to the word: authentic.

I posted all the way through my last trimester, continuing on at the gym five times a week, and the interest in my story only grew as my pregnancy progressed. People said it inspired them, seeing me so determined as I worked out, barely twenty years old and filled with motivation. I launched my fledgling business with that $400 budget, investing my precious nest egg into creating some PDFs of workouts.

The idea was to do the concepts myself on my home computer then get a professional illustrator to create images of me working out. But wow, I seriously underestimated the challenge of trying to master Word and Photoshop! I'm not sure I slept much, but somehow I bumbled my way through – it's amazing what passion will do. You don't even seem to notice how hard you're working. More importantly, I knew, despite its amateurish beginnings, I had something saleable. Best of all, it was my own thing.

As the PDF orders kept coming, I kept sending them out. I was backing myself, even as some people still shook their heads. I kept my eye on the prize, kept doing what *I* loved because I knew I held the key. That old saying, 'If you love what you do, you'll never work a day in your life' never felt truer. Despite working harder than I'd ever worked before, somehow I felt as if I was flying. Isn't it weird how you can turn things around, just by looking at them differently?

I didn't realise it at the time, but what I was really learning was *perspective*. Life is all about what you make it. Being pregnant and working out with my big belly gave me something authentic to share. There was nowhere to hide my bump, so I had no choice but to present the true me: the nature girl embracing life and on yet another adventure; the teenager using all the advice in those books; the uni student who blew her mind in a meditation class and never looked back. I was Tammy, the *real* Tammy, on display and unapologetically being myself. If you look back through my posts, you can see how my outward appearance has changed, and if you read my posts and listen to my podcast, you can see how my tastes and interests have changed, but who I truly am as a person on the inside has never changed. To this day, that honesty is the foundation of my business success.

What does 'authentic you' look like?

This exercise is fun because you can embrace all the weird and wonderful things about you! Not just from now, but across your life. Let's have a look through the years and pull out all your unique characteristics. Then let's see if you can embrace 'you' even more.

How would you describe yourself in primary school?

1. Things I loved to wear/eat: ....

....

....

2. Things I loved to say/do: ....

....

....

3. Things I was good at: ....

....

....

4. Words to describe me: ....

....

....

How would you describe yourself in high school?

1. Things I loved to wear/eat: ....

....

....

2. Things I loved to say/do: ....

....

....

3. Things I was good at: ....

....

....

4. Words to describe me: ....

....

....

How would you describe yourself now?

1. Things I love to wear/eat: ....

....

....

2. Things I love to say/do: ....

....

....

3. Things I am good at: ....

....

4. Words to describe me: ....

....

....

How would your closest friend/s describe you now?

1. Things I love to wear/eat: ....

....

....

2. Things I love to say/do: ....

....

....

3. Things I am good at: ....

....

....

4. Words to describe me: ....

....

....

Procrastination is, literally, a waste of time.

WORST-CASE SCENARIO

One thing I didn't expect when I started my business was how fast things would move. Looking back, it was pretty insane to open shop at the same time as having my son, Wolf. But at the time, I didn't think about it. Firstly, I didn't have time, but mostly, you don't think about things like that when you're super excited and jumping in, completely naive, but oh, so positive. Optimism works like blinkers on a horse. It keeps your focus on the track in front of you.

Personally, I think that's a good thing. So many amazing things in life might never have happened if we stopped to think about all the negatives. I'm not saying you shouldn't consider the pros and cons, but if we let fear hold us back, we'd never get anywhere. If you want to succeed, you have to ignore all the what ifs: *what if I can't sleep, what if I am kidding myself and this fails dismally?* You just have to keep going.

In the end, all that chatter is just fear talking. Unless it's going to make you sick or hurt someone, I think it's perfectly fine to ignore it. I mean, what's the worst that can happen – failure? So what! You can always start again.

That goes for absolutely any goal. Starting again = worst-case scenario. Once you take that fear away, you can make a start at anything. Fear can be paralysing which is the last thing you need. It leads to procrastination – which is, quite literally, a waste of time. And, in the beginning especially, time is something you can't afford to lose. You are going to need it more than anything else. It all flies by really, *really* fast.

*

For me, it felt like an overnight double-whammy. All of a sudden Wolf was born and I was starting this business from scratch. My days were jam-packed with sending out workout PDFs, looking after a newborn, getting in a gym session, and posting on my ever-growing Instagram account. I had *no* sleep and I'd never worked so hard in my life. Even though it might sound like hell, I loved every minute of it.

Maybe I was a bit manic from lack of sleep, but when you love what you do, it isn't work. And for me, motherhood was the best, most incredible thing. I think I was on a post-baby high, working from home, my family popping in and out. I was making my dreams come true, cocooned inside a happy mummy bubble – beyond perfect from my point of view. Obstacles and stress fade when you're wrapped in such a warm blanket of love.

Yes there were challenges, and more to come – mostly lack of sleep and all the worries that come with having your first baby. Looking back though, I wouldn't change any of it. I had to do what I had to do to make the business happen and there was *no way* I was going to miss a thing when it came to Wolf. Lack of sleep and worry seemed small prices to pay.

Besides, I was taught a long time ago by my step-dad never to complain. I truly believe in turning your face towards the sun (or rain), because everything in life is here for you to experience and grow from, both good and bad. If you let the rain stop you, or find yourself too nervous or afraid to even start, you're depriving yourself of some of the best moments ever, and the opportunity to flourish. And you'll never have those big moments in the sun

I was always taught to NEVER complain. You either work to change the situation, or if it's something you can't change, what's the use in complaining, right? That advice always resonated deeply with me, so I thought I'd share it with you guys too. ✌️ if you don't give yourself the chance to experience them. So jump in and experience it all. Things have a way of working themselves out in the end.

As they did, somehow, for me. I kept showing up, Wolf kept growing, and the cashflow into the business kept growing too. I was starting to make money from Instagram promotions as well, enough to fund my first investment, the next, very big step on the road to my dream: the Tammy Fit app. But just as I thought I had found my feet and gained some stability, seemingly overnight, everything, and I mean *everything*, changed.

How to get unstuck

Do you want to do something, but feel too worried to start? Maybe there are challenges in your way, such as lack of money or time, or maybe you're just feeling lazy. But for whatever reason, you find yourself procrastinating. Here's an exercise that may help kickstart things and get you moving. First, write down your goal (what you want). Then add the best- and worst-possible outcomes. Often, once you've written out your fears, you'll realise they are not so scary after all and you no longer have a reason to hold back. If you do discover something that truly worries you, try to put into perspective how likely it is to happen. Also look to the best-case scenario and allow its possibility to propel you forward.

What I want	Worst-case scenario and what I'd do then	Best-case scenario and how I would feel
To win the next club race.	I fall off my bike and injure myself. I take a month off to recover – why not make it a holiday!	I win the race, win some wine and drink it with friends. I feel like a champion!

RELATIONSHIPS

If you've looked at my social channels, you'd know that my family and relationships mean *everything* to me. They are my number one priority – what drives me forward and gives me strength. They're also my Achilles heel, as trolls use them to take advantage of me.

There's nothing worse than having people you love being used, especially your kids. It's made me pretty private and very wary about oversharing, though my life on social media may sometimes appear otherwise. That said, I understand that trolling and media intrusion comes with the business life I've chosen. I truly do appreciate all my followers and the life I get to lead. I accept that both the good and bad is all part of the experience.

Working out how best to balance my business success and personal life may be the biggest challenge I've faced. It's been tough at times, and I still don't have all the answers, but I'm getting there. As with everything I do, I know that even in the hard times, the secret is to get up and get moving. Showing up to my work and for my family is how I make every day count.

*

Once I'd started my fitness journey and seen the success of the PDF, I knew that Tammy Fit, the app, was *the* big goal. I was using a lot of different apps for different things and could see myself how convenient they were. It made sense that people would want a one-stop health and fitness hub that they could carry around in their pocket.

I planned for it to be the best app ever and have absolutely *everything*: meals, workouts, yoga, meditation, the lot. I also decided to give it its own Instagram account, so it could become its own brand – an extension of myself, yet standalone. There was so much involved in creating, launching and sustaining it, in some ways it was like having another child.

At that point, though, *no-one* was doing fitness apps so there was no mapped path to follow. This made it feel a bit risky. But I looked around. By now, a few original Instagrammers had over a million followers, yet they still weren't tapping into their captured market potential. I had seen success with my PDF and knew I could transform it into something bigger. It was time to show up.

Building the app would cost nearly every cent I'd made from the PDFs and promotional earnings, but I was convinced of its potential. One of the things I'd learnt in my step-dad's library was: to make money, you need to spend money. *Capitalise, reinvest, grow.*

I took a leap of faith. I handed over all my hard-earned cash and, after a lot of work behind the scenes, Tammy Fit was born. My followers already loved my health and fitness plans, so I knew they would love the app. To grow, I simply needed more followers. Once they liked what they saw and felt part of this amazing community, I knew they would want in. Tammy Fit would make them feel good and healthier too. For some, it might even be life-changing, as health and fitness had been for me.

My passion and conviction for changing people's lives drove me on. Despite many sleepless nights looking after baby Wolf,

I knew in my heart that pushing on was the only option. Driven by unshakeable belief, I applied consistent effort and watched the numbers grow. Success began to snowball and suddenly *I* was the one with over a million social media followers. Soon after, a million people had downloaded my app.

They came from all over the world. Success in the US and UK was exciting enough, but I didn't expect big numbers from places like Spain or Portugal. People were asking for translations in multiple languages.

It was all so huge, I could barely take it in. The girl from Currumbin Valley still vividly recalled arriving in Singapore, walking into that house and that library and having her mind blown. This was yet another pinch-me moment. For the first time, I had a lot of money. People were calling me an 'overnight' success! But before I'd had a chance to fully appreciate how far I'd come, my world took another grand twist. I fell pregnant with my daughter, Saskia.

At this point, Wolf was just six months old, I had a million-dollar business on my hands and I was only twenty-one years old. Suddenly it all felt very big and *very* overwhelming. My business-empire-building efforts and my newborn work baby, Tammy Fit, were going to have to fit in alongside raising two tiny, beautiful humans. I was determined to be a full-time hands-on mum and to keep growing the app and business that bore my name. They were important to me and I knew no-one could love them more. It made sense that I should bear full responsibility for their success. I resolved to do it all.

Soon I would learn my hardest lesson. And more than one relationship was going to fall apart.

Risky business
can be a risky
<3 business.

HOW MUCH IS TOO MUCH?

Trying to achieve too much at once can be exhausting, but at the same time, it's also important to make the most of your opportunities. When you start out as an entrepreneur, you spend a lot of your days working non-stop but only making incremental progress. So at a certain point, when everything finally clicks and success arrives, it feels impossible – plain wrong – to slow down. If hard work and constant effort got you here, then taking your foot off the accelerator is counterintuitive.

Sounds like a good problem to have, and it is, but it's also very tricky. Running your own business is risky and I'm not just talking about the money side of things. It's a risk at the heart level too, because your decisions impact your loved ones. When you commit to something time-consuming and high pressured, you're taking that on for the people who care about you too. How you let the pressure affect you, affects them as well.

*

I didn't see any point in slowing down during my second pregnancy, any more than my first. Again, people followed my journey – in far larger numbers this time. I was on a high from all the success and the thrill of having another baby. Feeling energised and more motivated than ever, soon after Saskia was born, I decided to launch my second big business: Saski – an international clothing line, named after my beautiful baby girl.

Attempting this with a newborn, a toddler and an existing business might sound crazy, but for me it was the logical next step. I was living in activewear and promoting fitness on a massive scale and I *love* fashion, so designing and selling my own brand felt like a no-brainer. Why wear other people's lines when I could wear my own? A lot of people thought I was taking on way too much, but I refused to listen. Instead, I used their negativity to fuel me.

As a social influencer, wearing someone else's brand can be restrictive. You're often committed to wearing outfits whether you like them or not and posting about them at certain times. For me, that felt like having a boss ordering you about – several bosses, in fact – and I'd gone into my own business to *avoid* all that. Once again, it was time to show up.

There was only one problem: I had no idea how to go about it. Though I'd learnt a lot from my fashion guru sister Emilee, and people seemed to like my style, I still had a lot to learn. My gut instinct was telling me this would work, but even *I* knew I couldn't take on a second huge business on my own! Finally, I asked for help.

My sister Amy was the perfect choice. She has a very different brain to mine – business-oriented and very organised – which complements my big-picture, creative thinking perfectly. I knew she would be the ideal person to manage Saski for me and make it something amazing. Fortunately, she agreed. I felt so relieved and excited. Not only did I have a business ally, I had my sister, one of my closest friends, by my side.

I know everyone says don't work with family, but I figured, who can you trust *more*? By then I'd had my fair share of people trying to get close to me purely because I was successful. It's such a strange and awful feeling, to have others try to leech off you and take advantage. I needed Amy not only for her business acumen but for her protection and support. Trust. I was beginning to learn just how important that is.

How to ask for help

Are you the kind of person who finds it hard to ask for help? Or do you do the opposite and lean too hard on others because you're not confident in doing things yourself? I believe trust starts with trusting yourself first, then choosing wisely when trusting others. This exercise is all about enlisting support to achieve a goal.

Something I want to achieve	How I am trusting and believing in myself to get this done	Who I am entrusting to help and support me	How I'm going to feel once I achieve it

A working
relationship
trumps a hard
work relationship.

WHEN IT WORKS . . . AND WHEN IT DOESN'T

Relationships are everything. You can't take your money with you, so who loves you at the end is all that really matters. Who's going to show up for you when you have nothing left to give? Or if you've made a terrible mistake? Who's going to make you laugh, reminiscing about the times that made you both happy? Who's going to remind you of all you've achieved, tell you how proud they are, say thank you?

It's tough balancing your relationships with putting maximum effort into your career and your achievements. How can someone be proud of you, if all you've done is laze around watching Netflix? How can you make memories on an unforgettable trip if you haven't earnt the money to travel? And just because you love someone, doesn't mean you should do everything together.

We need different companions for different reasons. And sometimes, the best partner is yourself. Your heartthrob may not be the best financial advisor; your grandma, perhaps not the best prom date. There's influence, authority and expertise on the one hand; passion, celebration and experimentation on the other. Figuring out who your best wing person is for any given adventure is part of the fun. Often it's based on what you want from the moment. Almost always, there are boundaries to consider.

When those roles become entwined, say, if your boss becomes your boyfriend, or your sister becomes your colleague, things are bound to get tricky. As with any relationship, working out the new dynamics takes effort. Sometimes, things go pear-shaped, as I was about to find out.

*

Working with Amy was wonderful at first. She worked with me from home, my babies by my side, as we formulated my very first clothing line. It was hectic, as you can imagine, but also such a buzz, and so much fun.

Our different brains worked in perfect tandem to produce and launch Saski. We were an awesome team, yet over time, things got tense. We were on top of each other every day and our lifelong roles as sisters (Amy, older and in charge) versus our work roles (me, as boss), led to conflict. It was really starting to affect our relationship, to the point where we had to decide what was more important: working together or our connection as sisters.

We found out the hard way that long-established roles in your personal life don't always suit the workplace. It's not that you shouldn't work with family, it's that you need to find a way to make it work. Usually things need to change, on one level or another. And if that's impossible, then the solution is clear: let the working relationship go.

While our differences worked well to establish Saski, over time it became obvious that they would cause problems. In the beginning it was brilliant – perfect in fact, and after the launch, I made her general manager. But we then started bickering. You can give each other whatever role or job title you like, but ultimately, Amy will always be my big sister. I adore her for that, but in the workplace, it was hard for us to switch roles. In the end, we realised that if we wanted to maintain our relationship, she would have to leave Saski. Fortunately, we both agree that our

I always get asked how I stay so positive all the time. While I'm a very positive, happy person & love my life so, so much, I'm also human & like everyone else have bad days, go through different phases and stages of life, face tough situations & raw emotions. But it's the small habits and the little things you practise daily that can make the biggest difference. A bad day doesn't mean a bad life. Every storm will pass. ☁

sister bond is more important than anything, so while there were some tough conversations and heartfelt emotions at the time, we worked through them and are now closer than ever.

Amy still works with Tammy Fit and does a brilliant job as she's always done. As the app is very much a separate entity, this definitely suits us better. A *working* relationship trumps a *hard work* relationship every time.

Changing a relationship dynamic

Maybe your relationship needs boundaries, maybe it needs to adapt, or maybe it should pivot to something entirely new. As wisdom dictates, nothing is more important than the people you love, so approach this as if you were ninety and looking back on your life. What advice would ninety-year-old you give you about the relationship?

Dear me . . .

....

....

....

....

....

You're not perfect – you never were and you never will be, and that's perfectly okay.

BEYOND BEING PERFECT

Parenting a child is one of the biggest, most fun and most challenging relationships you can have. My life is so much richer for being a mum. However, before I could truly enjoy it, I had one massive lesson to learn: I had to let go of 'mother guilt'.

It's only natural to become obsessed with our babies. No-one can possibly prepare you for how you'll feel when you first meet that little human. 'Love' doesn't even come close, it's too small a word for that all-encompassing feeling of needing to protect them at all costs. *I would do anything – I don't need sleep ever again, they are so incredible and cute and perfect, my heart literally hurts.* We want to do every possible thing we can for them, but being a nurturer is full-on and full-time. It's easy to neglect yourself, but if you don't nurture yourself too, it will just get harder and harder. That baby needs you to look after yourself. It's not selfish, it's logical. And it's kind.

*

I know mum guilt comes with the territory, but it can be really tough to deal with. When the kids were newborns, it was particularly bad for me. 'You can't always be there, Tammy,' my family tried to tell me. 'You can't always be perfect.' *I know,*

Mother /ˈmʌðə/ 🌸 👾
a person who loves
unconditionally, a protector,
a nourisher, someone that
does anything to put another's
happiness & wellbeing ahead of
their own. One whose heart no
longer beats for themself, but
for another.

*I know, but also . . . **no!** Maybe other people can't, but I can! In fact, I am, see?*

My commitment to the kids was all about being everything for them, all the time. My partner was busy when the babies were born, so it was pretty much all down to me. When Wolf and Sass were little, I didn't have any employees and I didn't have a nanny, which suited me fine. I didn't *want* any help. Maternal instinct + my natural-born stubbornness was a potent combination. I was determined to do it all by myself.

Unsurprisingly, I soon started feeling overwhelmed . . . to the point where I couldn't handle it. Thankfully, the Hembrow clan were lining up to help me. The hardest thing was teaching myself to let them. I'm not gonna lie – it was tough. It's difficult to trust others when it comes to your kids, even your own family, because you're letting them look after your heart! But the old saying is true: it really does take a village to raise a child.

On top of the physical effort of caring, being a mum brings many challenges. Until you're in it, you don't realise just how killer a lack of sleep is. There's a truckload of hormones running around in your body as well. For first-time mums, there's also the fact you're learning to do something entirely new and unfamiliar with no proper training. And someone's life depends on it – on *you*. It's a lot.

Not to mention that most of us are still trying to maintain a regular life of work, health and social commitments. Often, others are depending on you too. In my case, I was trying to be a partner, a friend, a sister, a daughter and, hugest of all, a boss – trying to be everything for everyone and also be everywhere all at once. It took me a long time to admit that I am just one person. **One.** It took me a long time to realise that the best way to give my babies the best life possible was to let other people help.

I'd quickly grown comfortable being the one in charge, the one responsible for my own success or failure. I felt uneasy letting others in. It took of lot of reverse-thinking to realise that allowing people to help was kinder than shutting them out. I've never wanted to be a burden, but watching me struggle was hard on those who care about me. Allowing them to help was the most gracious thing I could do.

It was selfish, I realised, to keep them at arm's length and only allow them to be part of my life in ways that I dictated. Opening myself up and letting people count in *all* the ways that mattered was scary, yes – it makes you vulnerable – but ultimately, so rewarding. Your relationships become richer and fuller. But it requires trust. Being 'good' at relationships means allowing relationships to flow both ways, give-and-take. So . . . I learnt how to delegate and trust the people closest to me to help – and that's how I was able to grow my businesses *and* be a good mum. I wouldn't have been able to do either of those things if I hadn't softened. I had to let go to some degree. I had to amend the commitment to being 'everything for them' to being 'everything for them – *with help*'.

People ask, 'How do you have it all?' I don't have it all, I have help. And love. Which *is* what I define as all.

I found it really difficult to admit I needed it at the start. Being independent and headstrong is what helps you launch global businesses. But it doesn't always help you raise a family. So I changed, in an effort to become the best version of myself. You can't be that if you're stressed and worried.

Add in self-care

Are you making sure there's also some 'me time' among all that 'mum time'? Can you let people in to help so you can nurture you too?

1. What can you do in the morning to care for yourself emotionally/physically/spiritually?

....

....

2. What can you do in the afternoon to care for yourself emotionally/physically/spiritually?

....

....

3. What can you do in the evening to care for yourself emotionally/physically/spiritually?

....

....

4. What can you do on weekends to care for yourself emotionally/physically/spiritually?

....

....

You can't start
again without an
ending.

BEND OR BREAK

Being the best version of yourself is easy when life is good. It's much harder when times get tough, and the worst when your support person is at the centre of the heartbreak. When your biggest relationship is disintegrating, who else can help you to make sense of things? Because every time you try to talk to *them*, things fall further apart. Of *course* there's love there. And kids involved too. So you try again and again, as hard as you can, to make it work. Until it doesn't.

For a long time, feeling guilty about the inevitable fallout stopped me from taking the action I knew my partner and I needed. When things don't work out, many people find it hard not to blame themselves. And sure, I'm all for accountability. But in these situations, it's not really your fault, or the other person's fault either – it's the relationship. The relationship failed, not you. Not one, not the other, but your combination.

In order to move on, you need that understanding. You have to do it for your kids. Because they need you to be kind to yourself in that moment, more than ever.

*

My partner and I broke up when Wolf and Sass were toddlers. It took everything within me to see it as a failed relationship, not a 'failed Tammy', and keep going. My parents had split up when I was young and I hated the idea of becoming a single mum. Although I'd become better at asking for help, the guilt made me want to become a supermum. I told myself I had to do it all, to *be* it all. There's no mother guilt like broken-relationship mother guilt. And desperation that your kids won't be sad because of it.

Breaking up with Wolf and Saskia's dad was the hardest thing I'd ever gone through. And I was devastated when it happened *again* after having my third baby, Posy. Ultimately, her dad and I just weren't meant to be. I never, ever wanted that kind of heartbreak, not for any of us. When you commit to love, your heart makes the choice. When you have children together, the choice to love is made for you again. I didn't want the relationships I had with my children's fathers to change and I didn't want the commitment to either of them to come to an end.

Yet no matter how much you might want a relationship to keep working, some things are beyond your control. While some connections can bend and morph, others break in the process. I struggled with that reality. As the child of divorced parents, I always wanted a strong and stable family life for my children. My parents didn't get along and fought a lot – to the point that my sisters and I don't know how they were ever together. So when I had my first two kids, I was determined to make the relationship with their father work. We were young, however, and people change. We grew in opposite directions.

What do you do when your home life isn't the happy dream your heart chose for you? Do you stay together 'for the kids'? The longer we stayed together, the more unhappy our home became and I didn't want to warp my kids' idea of what a healthy relationship looks like. In the end, it was a straightforward decision: do what was best for my home and my children. Do what was best for us all.

I'm not going to go into the ins and outs of our relationship, obviously we're human, we're not perfect. We have ups and downs like everybody else . . .
I just wanted to let you guys know that we're not currently together. I don't want people to think that we just gave up. Like most people would know, there's a lot more to it when it comes to relationships – they're very complex. We love each other very much and we're always going to be a family no matter what. Our kids come first, their health and their happiness are always going to be my number one priority.

There are no new beginnings without endings, but getting to that point can seem impossible. It does end, eventually. After some time, you feel like you again. You find a new way to make things work. Life evolves.

Free up your tomorrow

Do you need to bring an end to something in your life? Maybe you're stuck in a job you hate, or living too far from friends and family, or carrying a loan you can't afford because 'one day' it'll be worth it. Perhaps, like I did, you know in your heart a relationship has to end.

It may be the hardest thing you have to do, but when it's done, it's done. What you can get done today, will free up tomorrow. And every day after that. Taking that tough step will clear a new way forward. Even taking a moment to think things through can help. Here's an exercise to get you started.

If I could change one thing it would be:

....

I'm not doing it because:

....

Something I could do about it is:

....

How would I feel if it were done?

....

The only thing
you can control
is your reaction.

STICKS AND STONES

When you make a big life-changing decision, like breaking up with your partner, people will talk. Even if they don't say it to your face, they're still going to say it. People take sides and loyalties are tested. It hurts to lose some people from your corner.

I remember a friend saying to me that she took forever to break up with her long-term partner because she didn't want to lose his family. I get that. As anyone who's been through it will tell you, you quickly learn who your friends are. Often you lose people you've become close with because that's how loyalties lie. It's extra hard when your heart is breaking for your kids and you're vulnerable. Harder still, when you're in the spotlight.

*

One of the most difficult parts of being a public figure is that people make assumptions about you and can be very vocal in their opinions. I know it comes with the territory and that this same attention has created my success. I am grateful for that every single day. That doesn't mean it's been easy to handle going through very painful, very public break-ups – twice.

People had a lot to say about it. *What's wrong with you?* they said. *You've failed again. Why can't you keep a man? Why don't you think of the children?*

They don't know what happens in private – they only know what they see in the media, mostly driven by headlines and clickbait. I had to learn that you can't control the criticism being flung your way. Haters gonna hate and you have to shake it off. The only thing you can control is how you choose to show up, how you *react*. That means filtering out the opinions of others and focusing on what works for you, your family and your business.

Are there times when I look back at my relationships and wonder where things went wrong? Of course. Has it made me wary of starting another relationship and going through this again? Absolutely. But I have learnt and grown a lot through my past relationships and I trust that this will bring better times ahead.

Break-ups equate to broken hearts and I do grieve losing what was good. There is regret, there is pain, but there is acceptance too. I made the decision to leave both my partners because, in the end, the bad outweighed the good. However, the details of my break-ups will forever remain behind closed doors. I made a pact with myself never to speak negatively about either of them in public and I've kept it. I stand by my decision to remain silent, although I do admit to crying on my sisters' shoulders every now and again!

What's the point in the whole he said/she said thing? I posted a short break-up announcement and that was all I was willing to say about it because what else *is* there to say? Break-ups suck. They're hard for everyone. But as we've all moved on, I'm grateful we've found a way to make things work. Though those times were some of the hardest I've ever been through, they're done. Although I felt like I would at the time, I didn't break.

How much do others' opinions affect you?

My sisters say I have a thick skin, a survival mechanism developed during childhood. Resilience is built, but it can also be a heavy armour to carry. I had to learn to unload a lot of that in order to let people in. Rather than shield yourself, listen to your inner cheer squad. Develop positive, self-affirming thoughts and ignore the insults from others.

Here are some powerful words. Circle the ones you think are true about you, then pick your top three. Next time someone tries to tell you something negative about yourself, remember: *you know who you are.*

- encouraging
- diplomatic
- thoughtful
- generous
- happy
- kind
- reliable
- loyal
- protective

- hard-working
- creative
- compassionate
- optimistic
- persevering
- smart
- talented
- loving
- fun

Life is ever-changing.

LOVING YOUR WAY ONWARDS AND UPWARDS

When relationships end or you go through a big crisis there's one thing you'll need more than anything: self-love. It is vital to give yourself plenty of compassion. These days, I use this as my armour.

All those positive words and reminders we just worked through are a way of re-programming yourself. What you believe is what you become, so self-talk really matters. It's more than just confidence – it's how you think about yourself, which ultimately affects how you behave in the world. Your 'self-relationship' is the most important relationship of all because it affects everything you experience.

Another thing that helps me stay calm during a crisis is knowing that life is ever-changing. The sun rises, the sun sets. This morning is sunny, yesterday was rainy. You were hungry, now you're full. Soon you'll be hungry again. It's nature's law that everything is always changing: the seasons, the weather. You. No matter how crappy a state you're in, this too shall pass. It must. It's nature's law.

*

Having my big sisters by my side has made my life what it is. To have someone you can trust, no matter what. They have wiped away my tears many times and been there cheering at every success. Being able to raise our babies beside one another means the world. It's an unbreakable bond. 🫶

A while after each of my break-ups, we eventually created new routines. Once the dust had settled and we'd all found our new 'normal', life moved on for me and my little family. Something else became clear too: when you hit rock bottom there's only one place to go – up!

I've learnt that positivity and resilience aren't so much personality traits as habits. It comes back to that programming thing. If you catch yourself thinking negatively, flip it around. It's up to you how you choose to see things. Like attracts like, so if you choose to focus on the negatives, then that is all you will see. The same principle applies when you focus on the positives.

When I was going through my break-ups, I found it hard at first to be positive about anything. Once I switched my focus from thinking about how I'd 'failed' at two relationships to realising the good things that had come from them – three beautiful, healthy babies, greater insight into myself, and so much more – I felt more empowered. It isn't easy to start, but developing a positive mindset is a bit like working out: if you keep strengthening that 'muscle' it will get stronger.

And of course, all this is much easier to do when you have support. Try to surround yourself with people who have your best interests at heart. Love will get you through this, both self-love and the love from them. I am incredibly fortunate in that I have beautiful parents and siblings who always get me through. Whenever I go through something tough, I lean on them. They keep me strong. I need to be that as a mother, and as a business leader too. A lot of people depend on me, no matter what kind of personal crisis I'm going through. I could see that as a whole heap of pressure or I can flip that thinking and see myself as incredibly lucky because the people who love me are always there.

'Doing it all' doesn't mean 'doing it all on my own'. Aside from my sisters and family, I have an incredible group of people around me at work. Delegating used to be as hard for me at work as it was at home. When I first started my businesses I wanted to do *everything* myself and have full control, but that just wore me down. Eventually I had to trust other people to help me there too. I now have the most wonderful team and employees. I couldn't do any of it without them.

Your people

When the going gets tough, you may feel vulnerable admitting you need help, but that's when relationships with family, friends and colleagues can grow to next level. Whether for now or in the future, think about the people in your life who are there for you in tough times, and equally, those you have supported. Write down their names and don't be shy to turn to them in good times and bad. If you don't feel confident with that list right now, what could you do to find new people or start strengthening those existing relationships today, so that they stand strong tomorrow?

My people:

....

....

....

....

....

....

One true friend
is true wealth.

OH-SO-PRECIOUS TRUST

I've talked about relationships with family, partners and colleagues, but aside from my sisters, I haven't talked about friendship. You might be one of those people who has so many friends you need a massive venue for any kind of party, the person who can't walk through a shopping centre without stopping to talk to half a dozen people and whom everyone seems to know. According to Dale Carnegie you're a success. In his book *How To Win Friends and Influence People*, he suggests you should be like the family dog when it comes to making friends – because everyone loves a dog, right? So wag your tail, be happy to see people, have no judgement. I love that idea, but for me, life is a bit different.

*

I'd love a wider circle of friends, but one of the big prices I've paid for my success is having my trust eroded by people wanting friendship for the wrong reasons. As a social influencer, people try to leech off you and there's another weird thing that happens: they want to steal your energy. This happens a lot with people who get attention or are in the spotlight – look at the lead singer of a band, or that kid who is super popular at school or good at sport. People want to be like them, and if they can't, they want to bask in their light.

It's magnified in online social circles. Profiles get boosted by connections, so some people just want to be *seen* as a friend rather than be one. This makes me wary of 'false friends' who are only in it to get something out of it. At the opposite end of the scale is the true friend. A real friend will be there when crap goes down, when people are pointing at you like some witch being led through the town square, when your light has lost its lustre. In those moments, having just *one* true friend is true wealth. They are worth more than all those fair-weather friends combined because they truly love you, no matter what.

My best friend Bella is one such person. I've been friends with her since the ninth grade. She's now the general manager of Saski which means I get to see her nearly every day. There's no other friendship like a long-term friendship; no-one else shares the same bond. Bella knows me inside out and we have been through a lot together. She is especially precious to me, because, although I made friends from all over the world at my international school in Singapore, I lost touch with most of them when I moved back to Australia.

I've kept a handful of other friends since school, and several of them work with me. I'm actually friends with all my employees – *real* friends – which is pretty awesome. It's another part of the reason why work doesn't really feel like work: I consider my employees part of the family. We have so much fun together and often organise social work outings with both the Tammy Fit and Saski teams combined. I'm so lucky that way.

It's easy to be overwhelmed in your life but friendship, as in *true* friendship, is a sacred thing. My advice is to make your true friends a priority. I know I haven't always done that, but I'm incredibly lucky that they've stood by me, regardless. These days, I don't take true friends for granted. If you've managed to hang on to a friendship long term, treasure it. It really is true wealth.

Tell them you care

Why do we wait until we're writing a birthday card to tell a friend we value and love them? Since they enrich our lives so much, I believe a true friend deserves more. This activity suggestion is a heart-warming one that runs both ways. Think of it as a 'just because' message, a non-birthday gift for the one you love.

Choose whichever writing method works for you: card, pen and paper or DM, then use the template below to create your own heartfelt message:

I wanted to tell you .... because

you are .... When I think back to

.... it makes me feel ....

I am so grateful to have you in my life because

....

Life certainly didn't pan out the way I had planned in so many ways. And for that, I am grateful. ♡ Thanking God every day for giving me peace, for giving me strength, for giving me the sunrise & sunset & most of all for giving me my beautiful babies.

MOVEMENT

As I said at the beginning: sometimes it isn't easy to show up each day. In fact, some days I choose to show up for PJs, Netflix and the lounge, or lying round the pool! Most days, though, I'm on.

Committing to your big dreams starts by *doing*. You need to move! Simply putting one foot in front of the other can take you to amazing places. You never know what may unfold, but one thing is certain: it will offer new experiences. That's one of the nicest things about life – every day holds its own story.

I've built an entire career out of movement – and in more ways than one. Obviously Tammy Fit and Saski are all about exercise and health and fitness/activewear and fashion, but it's what's moving *beneath* that's the real driving force. Before you start to move *physically*, you need to start by moving *mentally*.

I use my mind to overcome procrastination, to remind me how good a habit feels, to push me out of bed. Some of my best days have begun with ho-hum mornings. Debating whether to be bothered, my brain jumps in, *Yep, be bothered!* I know that once I get going, I'll soon be feeling fantastic from my workout and enjoying my day. If you lack motivation, get up and get moving. Motivation will follow.

I've been feeling less than
motivated in the gym this week,
but I will continue to show up.
And I will continue to give it my
all. It's not always easy but I make
myself find time even on the
busiest of days running around
after my kids and back and forth
in meetings/work. Why? Because
life is a continuous journey of
growth and self-development
for me, and my health is an
important aspect of that. When
you stop making excuses and start
showing up, it becomes habit.

The bottom line is: *mindset is everything.* You can mentally train your mind in the same way you train your body in the gym. There are lots of ways to keep your 'mind workouts' fresh and strong. As with any training, consistency is key, because what you repeatedly tell yourself to be, is what you will eventually become.

A motivated mindset is programmable. I am going to let you in on all the things I've done and strategies I've employed to move my life forward in a positive way. And of course, being about movement, we'll get into the physical side of things too.

You are what
you eat, do
and think.

WHAT GOES IN COMES OUT

We've all heard the saying, 'You are what you eat.' It's truer to say that you are what you *do*, as in: eat, exercise, sleep. But even more importantly: you are what you *think*.

Just as you train your body with exercise, your thinking can also be drilled. As with any good program, it's as much about what you do, as what you don't. What you consume *and* what you avoid. One of the best ways to manage your mind is to be mindful of what you let in.

Think about how you feel when you see something tragic on the news. Now, think about how you feel when you're listening to one of your favourite songs. Totally different energy, right? Being selective about what goes into your brain is powerful. Reading is my go-to method and screentime is also a relaxing way to get some positive input. I listen to podcasts and audio-books too, which are so easy to fit in when you're driving, doing housework, travelling or exercising.

*

Those years in my step-dad's library left a lasting impression on me. I especially love reading books on personal development and always feel super motivated once I've finished one.

Even reading just a few pages can plant an idea that lasts the whole day! Not only is it a great way to get some positive input, it's also great value timewise. If you're sitting down with a cup of tea in the morning, why not jump into a quick motivational session via a book or podcast? It's easy to fit in and super effective.

Here's a list of some inspirational books I've enjoyed over the years:

Atomic Habits by James Clear
How to Win Friends and Influence People by Dale Carnegie
Rich Dad Poor Dad by Robert Kiyosaki
Start With Why by Simon Sinek
Success Habits by Napoleon Hill
The 4-Hour Work Week by Timothy Ferriss
The 7 Habits of Highly Effective People by Stephen R. Covey
The Magic of Thinking Big by David Schwartz
The Power of Now by Eckhart Tolle
The Success Principles by Jack Canfield
Think and Grow Rich by Napoleon Hill

Many of these touch on the importance of cultivating gratitude. Being grateful for where I'm at and how far I've come motivates me to keep going when I'm feeling low. A powerful gratitude habit I often use is taking a few moments each morning and night to mentally list and appreciate all the people and things I am grateful for. It's like running a highlight reel of my favourite show through my mind. It always leaves me feeling uplifted and happy.

Motivation mindset exercise
Everyone is different and we all find unique ways to motivate ourselves, keep our mindset strong and follow through on our commitments to our dreams and goals. Take a moment to consider what helps *you* most, and how you might like to incorporate them more into your daily routine.

1. These are the books I want to read/podcasts I want to listen to/shows and movies I want to watch so I can plant more positive seeds:

....

....

....

....

2. These are the ways I will be practising gratitude to remind myself of all the good things in my life:

....

....

....

....

Mental & physical health go hand in hand 🤝. That is why I train. Everything is connected and I feel my best when I am consistently pushing, consistently training, consistently getting stronger.

What motivates
you makes you
stronger.

'GOOD' PUSHING

Figuring out when and how far and how hard to push yourself is a tricky one. Younger me would have said, 'Go hard at all costs to make your dreams come true!' But I've learnt that sometimes it's more important to take the pedal off the metal and change direction. You need to know your limits and focus on what's *really* important. If you're heading down the wrong path, your intuition will be sending you messages. Listen! Keep an honest account of what's happening both *to* you and *around* you, and check in with your inner self.

'Good' pushing is when it *feels* good. Pretty simple, I know – often the right answers are. You know your limits and, if you don't, your body will tell you. Or your brain. Stress and exhaustion aren't things you can ignore forever. Good pushing is when you're still motivated by the push, when you're going that extra mile and you're proud of yourself because you're kicking goals. When pushing is good, it's *powerful*. You feel motivated, invincible, proud of yourself and inspired! This is when it's worth pushing yourself to your limits.

'Bad' pushing, on the other hand, leaves you in a state of permanent exhaustion. You can barely decide what to eat for breakfast, let alone make sound business and personal decisions.

You won't feel like yourself and will have a semi-permanent, anxious sensation in your gut. Instinctively you'll know something is off, but if you're a Type-A personality like me, that might encourage you to push even harder. If things continue getting tougher, stop. If you've lost your mojo and motivation, stop. Ask yourself, *How long has this been going on?* If it's been longer than a few weeks, something's not right. Take a moment, take stock and re-evaluate.

Motivation is key here. The difference is, have you been a bit out of whack for a day or two, or have you been consistently off kilter for weeks? Your motivation should make you feel stronger, as if you could conquer the world.

*

When you know what you're showing up for, you know it's worth it. My kids are a huge motivation for me. They inspire pretty much everything I do. I want to help them build the best lives ever and I want to set a great example of how to live my best life while I'm at it.

This big-picture thinking allows me to focus less on the obstacles I face and more on the goals ahead. My kids are my true reason for pushing through. My happiness comes back to them, so I have photos of them and drawings and cards they've made in places where I can see them every day, to keep them front of mind. When your work is inspired at the heart level, you can achieve *anything* – and my kids are completely and utterly my heart.

I'm also motivated to do this for myself. I've always been committed to personal growth and development. What's the point of being here otherwise? Along the way, I've learnt that good pushing can be a bit tricky and involves more than just moving out of your comfort zone – you have to get *comfortable* with being *uncomfortable*. Embrace that hard thing.

One thing that helps me meet those challenges head on is

I honestly love mornings so, so, so much. The start of a new day, the sunrise, the possibilities, the tiny sleepy faces I get to wake up to. Just everything. And I love the moments of quiet 'me time' before the school morning rush and a busy work day.

describing the act as *daring*. I'm inspired by all the women who've fought for change. Who dares, wins.

Once you've conquered that first hill, it gets easier after that – not because it gets *physically* easier, but because you know what you're in for and can set your mind to the task. For example, when I train, it's never easy, and it never gets easier. If it does, I know I'm not pushing myself enough. But I also know the rewards that will follow and, because I know that in advance, it's easier to show up.

It's much, much harder to leap into the unknown and do things that you aren't comfortable or familiar with. For me, one of those big things was public appearances. For someone in the spotlight I am an oddity because I really *am* shy and hate public speaking. I get hot and flustered and nervous. At first, it was almost too much for me to handle. But I had to. My career choice as an influencer made it impossible for me to avoid.

I had to get comfortable with being uncomfortable. I had to do some good pushing. When I felt stuck, I leant into my motivation. Of all the things I've achieved, forcing myself to take on public speaking, feeling the discomfort and doing it anyway, is one of my proudest accomplishments.

Having felt how powerful discomfort is, these days, I seek it out! There's growth in feeling the fear and pushing through it because you feel so proud of yourself when you do. When a challenge lies ahead, I often take time to reflect on that. It gives me motivation to proceed. Doing the easy things in life is easy, doing the hard things is growth.

Get motivated

Do you have anything or anyone that motivates you to achieve more? Are there 'uncomfortable' things blocking your way? Thinking about that, tap into your inner strength as you answer the prompts below.

Thing I want to do	Who or what motivates me	What might be blocking me	How can I be daring and do it anyway

Are you going to
be the victim or
the creator?

A WONDERFULLY STRUCTURED ROUTINE

For some it may sound boring, but I love structure and routine! Structure makes things happen and routine *keeps* them happening. Positive change. Moving forward. Sometimes establishing a working structure means shifting things around and freeing up space so that new stuff can occur. It's not all boring repetition. It can help us move mountains.

Everybody's unique and we all have our reasons for getting out of bed in the morning. We each have different lives to show up for, parts of which we love and other parts we'd like to change, such as a habit we're trying to break. We also have people we're showing up for, the ones who make everything worthwhile, who motivate us to be the best we can be. We want to have time for them, most of all.

What are you showing up for? Is your life how you dreamt it, or are your days spent doing things that bring you down? It's one thing to have plans, it's quite another to look at the reality of your everyday life. What does your daily routine look like – which elements would you like to keep, increase or change? If you're truly enjoying the life you've made and sharing it with those you love, showing up isn't a struggle, it's a total joy!

*

The gym will forever be my happy place. No kids (most of the time), no noise, no distractions. And I honestly don't know what I'd do without the @Tammyfitapp. I feel like I'm constantly on the go and at times it can get overwhelming, so having all my workouts in one place, not having to think about what I'm doing and really being able to switch off my mind is just 🤍.

If your everyday life is out of balance, here's your opportunity to consider fixing that. One of my favourite sayings is that there are two ways to approach life, as either the victim or the creator. Are you going to be a victim of the routine you're stuck in or are you going to create something better for yourself?

There have been times, over the years, when I found myself living a life I wasn't happy with. When this happens, the secret is to recognise and change it before it becomes ingrained. Everyone's routine gets out of whack now and then – notice when you start to feel overwhelmed, tired or resentful. Ask yourself whether it's a one-off or it has become a way of life? If it's in danger of becoming permanent and you don't like it, see what you can do to change it.

If you're feeling stuck or frustrated, chances are that your structure and routines have stopped working for you. You might be overdoing it in one sector of your life and underachieving in another. Maybe too much work and not enough play! Often parents put aside their own enjoyment to focus on work and caring, but then end up becoming grumpy, no-fun people. I'm sure that wasn't their intention for parenthood, I sure know it wasn't mine. If ever I find myself getting too serious, I make an effort to fix it. Kids are good for that.

Getting more organised doesn't have to be boring and predictable. Once you're done, it frees up time to do all the fun and exciting things! Life is about balance; how's yours?

Pick the low-hanging fruit

When it comes to being more organised and freeing up time to do more of what you enjoy, it pays to review your structure and routines.

1. Do you have a daily structure – an everyday basic schedule or plan?

2. Do you have a routines for each phase of the day: morning, daytime, evening?

Thinking about your current schedule and routines, are they:

1. A bit much. I never have time to stop and have a chat and always feel like I need to get on with the next thing.

2. Pretty good, actually. I get stuff done and there's still room for enjoyment!

3. What structure and routine? Life is for flying by the seat of my pants. If things are meant to get done, they will.

Sometimes all it takes is a small shift. Let's take a fresh look at how you spend your time.

What do you wish you had more time for?

....

....

Where do you waste time?

....

....

What could you move, adjust or add to your daily schedule to get more out of life?

....

....

Physically,
emotionally
and mentally,
working out is
the _best_.

MOVE, GLORIOUS MOVE!

The gym is the place where I can put everyday life on pause while I focus on building a healthier, stronger and fitter body. Mentally, I switch off from all distractions and responsibilities and can just be me. Exercising is so empowering – physically, emotionally and mentally. It gets your feel-good hormones flowing and enhances your sense of wellbeing. Exercise is the best way to start your day and I've never, ever regretted a workout. It's the one thing you have complete control over, while knowing it's doing you good.

I love motivational quotes and I'm a very visual person so when I started out I used to look at images of bodies I wanted to emulate and kept the images as screen savers. What keeps me motivated now is how I feel when I *don't* work out. I get tired and down and can't think straight. It's such a huge part of my life and the best thing about it is I can do it anywhere, anytime. And you can too.

*

When I first started exercising I lived with my sister Amy in a tiny flat. It was so small, the yoga mat took up all the floor space in the living room! I remember my sister walking in at

5 a.m. one morning and saying, 'Um, what are you doing?' There was hardly room to even step side-to-side properly, but I was so determined and motivated. I was addicted to it and I still am and that's a healthy thing because I also eat a lot. By eating well and moving lots, I keep myself in balance.

My body has changed a lot over the years. I've gone from super lean to softer, curvy and pregnant three times; from super fit to post-holiday a bit unfit, but I never stay away from the gym for long. People comment on my body all the time, and although my body is my job, the negativity still hurts. I used to get really upset but, like anything else, I learnt to grow an even thicker skin and got over it. I love to inspire people with their health and fitness, so I'm glad I've been able to show them my changing body. I plan to continue showing them – and showing up – no matter where I'm at in my journey.

When it comes to fitness, my main pieces of advice are:

1. It's your body, your journey and your decision as to how you want to look and feel. As long as that goal is healthy, go for it!

2. Engage the muscles correctly! The biggest mistake I see when people work out is that they don't focus on each individual muscle anywhere near enough. Visualise as you do weights. Picture that muscle contracting! It's my biggest tip.

3. Push yourself to the limit! You won't see results unless you give a hundred per cent.

4. Work on the whole body. It's important to have a stable core and work every muscle.

5. Exercise at the same time each day so that exercise becomes part of your routine. It's easier for me to be motivated early as I get distracted and sluggish later on, but you'll soon find what works best for you. The most important thing is *consistency*.

6. Be accountable . . . or have others hold you to account! It doesn't have to be self-driven, sometimes it's a good idea to

engage a coach to help you to remain focused on certain goals. Working out with friends is also a great motivator. You don't have to achieve things alone.

The secret to exercise success

Exercise 'success' comes down to what you view it as. Exactly what do you want to get out of this? Get clear on your goals and focus to get optimum results. It's worth reviewing these questions every three months to maintain progress.

1. What is your goal (specific to you + specific results)?

2. What do you need to improve about your workouts/exercise routine?

3. Are you ready to give this a hundred per cent?

4. What is your whole body plan?

5. How will you make sure you are consistent?

6. How will you hold yourself accountable?

My body has done so much for me, carrying my beautiful babies. Working out is my thank you. It's how I respect everything it's done and given me.

Sometimes
it's an excuse,
sometimes it's
a reason.

THANKS,
BUT NO

It's vital to push yourself, get moving and be consistent, but we're not machines. Most of the time I try not to let my mood dictate whether I exercise as often I find that once I move, my mood will lift. However, sometimes we just aren't feeling it for good reason. If you don't feel like working out, ask yourself what's *really* going on. Maybe you have a cold – is it so bad that rest and recovery is best or are you using that sniffle as an excuse to sleep in? Maybe there's something else, something deeper going on? Perhaps you're run down and pushing yourself too hard.

Asking yourself 'is it a *reason* or is it an *excuse*' works twofold. First, it's a good reality check – you're drilling down to the truth of the matter, which only you know. You may be able to kid yourself for a while, but in the end, it's no use lying to yourself because you're only letting yourself down. Pushing too hard, or not enough? Both can be equally detrimental, so get honest with yourself. Then make the change you need.

*

I can think of a million excuses for staying in bed at 5 a.m. and not working out. It's winter. It's cold. I'm tired! But none of them can compete with the main reason that I do get up and show up. For me, it's clear: getting out of bed and starting my day is all part of my big dream, my passion and my life's work – work that transforms other peoples' lives, too.

It's a humbling, wonderful privilege to help others become healthier and achieve their goals. It's also a big responsibility. An excuse like 'I'm tired' or 'I think I have a bit of a sniffle today' simply doesn't cut it. It's my job to inspire, motivate and uplift, while remaining honest about my moments of weakness, and 'being human' too. It's a balancing act, so when in doubt, I practise self-kindness. Often the kindest thing isn't to procrastinate or lie in bed, but to *move*. Get up and chase those dreams!

Another personal trainer told me once that the number one reason people find it hard to make working out a habit is that they *overthink* it. So instead of *overthinking*, his advice is to start *doing*. Put on your shoes, brush your teeth, throw on a hoodie and step outside! If you can't train until the kids are at school, get dressed for it anyway, and as soon as you've got them off, make a beeline for your workout. If after-work is most convenient for you, as soon as you knock off, head straight to the gym, no excuses. 'The doing is in the starting,' he says. So true.

Most of the time I get out of bed and do my early morning routine until I start feeling great, but it doesn't always work. All the mindset motivation in the world won't change a bad day and there's good reason for it: your body or mind is saying 'no'. I don't mean it's saying 'no' in a superficial, procrastinating kind of way, I mean, it's telling you something important at a deeper level – at times like that you need to listen. There's no use trying to chase your dream if it's causing you stress or unhappiness.

An equally important part of training is rest and recovery. Sometimes part of the process is stopping. I find if I really don't feel like showing up, or if I'm truly unmotivated or just not feeling myself, it's usually a sign that I need to take a break. So I do.

Check in with yourself

An excellent, quick way to help determine whether your excuse is legitimate or self-sabotage is this short self check-in. Don't let your shame demons get in the way; be honest with how you're feeling physically and emotionally and allow the right answer to come to the surface.

What is it I think I don't want to do?

....

....

How will I feel later about that?

....

....

There's one thing you'll always be awesome at: being you.

LOVING THE SKIN YOU'RE IN

I haven't always been fit. Or toned. Or the age I am, a mum, my current size. None of us has *always* been anything because we are all a work in progress. Body confidence is such a tricky thing, especially now, and I worry about my daughters and nieces in particular, because the pressure on them is going to be huge. It just keeps getting bigger, the whole 'perfection' ideal and, yes, you might be thinking that sounds a bit funny coming from me, but I've always had to work hard to keep in shape. I have been bigger, smaller, less fit, more fit – so many versions of me – but I have always loved the skin I'm in.

It's great to be fit and have good muscle tone, but it's so much more important to be 'fit' underneath it all, to have good *inner mental health*. If trying to chase an ideal of perfectionism is hurting you, then it will never be worth it. If exercise and a healthy life make you feel happy and energetic and wonderful about being you, then you're doing it for the right reasons and it's *definitely* worth it.

This is such a glass-half-full thing. For years, I've seen women (and men) frowning at the mirror in the gym, only seeing their flaws. I want to say to them, 'Hey, you're doing great!' If you love the life you're living and are happy with the effort you're making, then you've reached the ultimate goal. Look in that mirror and be proud of yourself.

*

I remember my mum being so positive about body confidence when we were growing up, even though our weights varied. My step-dad is a brilliant cook, so pasta in creamy sauce was often on the menu and there was no way I'd be saying no to that. My sisters and I have all been different sizes at various times, but Mum taught us to love our bodies. She always told us we were beautiful and I'm so thankful for that. So much of your self-confidence comes from the attitude you have towards yourself. And this is affected by the people around you, especially growing up.

High school can be a deadly black hole, especially when it comes to how much others' opinions affect your self-worth. I remember being hassled about my teeth and being called 'horsey' which really upset me. I was bullied in other ways too – at times physically. On one occasion, someone had their hands around my neck and another time my friend and I had our heads bashed together. Mum was such a protector, I didn't want to tell her about it – she'd have marched into the playground and demanded justice. Once a boy had to give my sister flowers for pushing her over!

Bullying is such sly, confidence-destroying behaviour, but it seems to me that, with or without it, everyone ends up with some kind of insecurity. But, as with any kind of exposure therapy, I've built up an immunity to bullying and I've certainly grown a thicker skin. I still don't understand why bullies do it, though. Why would anyone want to put someone down and make them feel bad about themselves just for fun? I guess they're projecting their own insecurities onto you, but it can still really hurt.

I despise bullying. But something we can do to protect our kids, each other and ourselves from it, is build each other up.

I've had the busiest week, guys. I've missed workouts, I've woken up late almost every day (I'm usually up at 5), I've forgotten things for the kids at school, run late to meetings. It can be so tempting to be hard on myself for all these little things but heyyy that's life. Not every week is perfect and you just gotta go with it and try again tomorrow.

If you think a compliment, say it out loud. There are endless opportunities to make someone feel good about themselves and build their self-confidence. It's such a gift to give them, and so, so important. I believe we should be our kids' number one cheer squad. I tell mine every day how funny, clever and beautiful they are. I want them to internalise positive self-talk so they can walk confidently out in the world, so that any negative comments will bounce straight off them.

You can compliment yourself too and prompt others to give you more. Every morning when you look in the mirror, think of something kind to say to yourself. Put post-it notes around the place to remind yourself how amazing you are and what you've already accomplished. The best is yet to come.

How much self-confidence do you really have?

List ten things you like about yourself on the outside and another ten things you like about yourself on the inside, and be *specific*. Not just, 'I have nice hair.' More like, 'I love my crazy curly hair because it matches my out-there personality.'

INSIDE

1. ....

2. ....

3. ....

4. ....

5. ....

6. ....

7. ....

8. ....

9. ....

10. ....

OUTSIDE

1. ....

2. ....

3. ....

4. ....

5. ....

6. ....

7. ....

8. ....

9. ....

10. ....

It isn't always
a workout,
sometimes
it's play.

PLAY TIME

Isn't it funny how often, as adults, we consider exercise a chore. Even if we like it, it's still one of those things we 'have to do'. We seem to have lost all the fun in it. Which is sad, when you think about it. As a kid, it wasn't like that. Exercise was playtime – skipping rope, chasing your friends around the oval, swinging along the monkey bars. Do that as an adult and people assume you're training for some gladiator show.

Exercise doesn't have to be about showing up at the gym or playing team sports. It isn't only about doing a class, or weights, or Pilates. Exercise is simply moving and loving the feeling of having your body respond to your commands. Ask anyone who has an injury or medical problem and they'll tell you not to take movement for granted. Sometimes our bodies are perfectly mobile, at other times, more limited. But they are designed to move, and as we learn to work with them, moving can feel good. It can be fun.

Whether it's walking round the shops, dancing to the beat, pushing your toddler on the swings, or doing your own vacuuming, every little move adds up. A good belly laugh and sex count too! Exercise is about actively embracing life. At its best, exercise is just moving – better still, playing.

*

One of the best things about being a mum has been rediscovering play. My kids and I do lots of crafts and cooking and playing games together, but the biggest playtime for us is just being active, indoors and out.

When we're inside, I love involving them if I'm doing a stretch or yoga session, or even just dancing around the house. They follow along and copy me and it's so much fun. As the daughter of a musician, music was a massive part of my childhood. It's equally huge in my household now, acting as a form of release and therapy. If I'm having a good day, I put on some music. If I'm having a bad day, I put on some music. I sing along loudly and I dance like no-one's watching. There's nothing more fun and stress-relieving than playing a favourite throwback track and dancing it out.

I consider the outdoors one giant playground. Living on the Gold Coast is paradise. We have endless beautiful beaches, rivers, rainforests and national parks where we can swim, hike, run and bike to our heart's content. Plus, we have water sports like kayaking and paddle boarding and surfing. In Queensland, it's easy to come out and play.

That said, I do travel a lot for work, and wherever I find myself, I make sure I get my exercise in. Wherever you live, I recommend getting physical as much as you can. There's so much joy to be had in embracing a healthy body. Better than any drug, moving gets the good vibes buzzing – and it's fun! Playtime isn't only for kids – it's for *everyone*.

More play!

Are you getting enough play in your day? You can burn a ton of calories by playing. Guess how many for each of the activities below.

Draw a line matching the activity with the amount of calories it burns for an hour:

Canoeing	450
Surfing	200
Disco dancing	300
Frisbee throwing	400
Hiking	400
Tree climbing	350
Hopscotch	200

[Answers: canoeing = 400, surfing = 200, disco dancing = 400, frisbee throwing = 200, hiking = 450, tree climbing = 300, hopscotch = 350]

Life is so cute & fun rn ⬤ 🍄
🌱 🌊 🌅 . Last night when the
moon started rising & we saw
the glowing red coming over the
horizon I literally SCREAMED and
we all ran down to the water's
edge. What a magical life we live.
🐌 🐌 🐌

NOURISHMENT

Nourishment means nutritious, delicious food for growth – of your body, mind, spirit and relationships. For life. My sisters constantly tease me that I never seem to stop eating. I love food! Healthy, nutritious and delicious. Mostly because it tastes good, but also for what it can give. Preparing food and feeding yourself and your loved ones is an act of care. In today's fast-paced world, it's easy to overlook that and reach for the quickest, most convenient bite. But if you can find time to make food, and sit for a moment to enjoy it – ideally if you can, share it – then it becomes so much more. Not only is it nourishing your body, it's nourishing your soul.

I know from experience that trying to be everything to everyone can cost too much. In order to give, you need to nurture and nourish yourself, and not put yourself last. When you grow up around ambition and success it can cultivate a drive within you to achieve the same – you can see that in my sisters and me. We followed in our step-dad's footsteps to become entrepreneurs, which takes a lot of drive and hard work. Less obvious is the need to balance that out with self-care and inner nourishment. You can't just expect be that driven and 'on' all the time, no matter how determined you are. I learnt that the hard way.

That said, it takes care, attention and effort to nurture tiny seeds. In the beginning, they need the perfect growing conditions to sprout. Only once you have carefully tended them through infancy do their roots grow strong enough to be self-sustaining. Being pregnant and with $400 to start a business meant I had to give it everything and more. Today, although I still work in it daily, the business flourishes without me having to do every last task. It has grown a trunk and branches and leaves which keep it strong through all seasons. It has spawned a second business and several ongoing ideas, all supported by staff. There are so many trees and saplings and new shoots, you could probably call my businesses a grove – not quite a forest, but we will get there eventually! All because the seed of an idea was nourished with the right care and attention from the get-go, and continues to receive the right attention to keep it performing.

From little things, big things grow – so long as they are nourished.

I have worked hard over the years and it has not always been smooth sailing trying to juggle it all. I am so lucky to have created businesses that I am very passionate about.

Every day you
build yourself
with the food
choices you
make.

FOOD CHOICES = YOU

I love food. I eat at least five times a day and every mouthful is a pleasure. But it wasn't always this way. When I was younger, I had quite an unhealthy relationship with food. I bounced from one extreme to the other, and though I knew it wasn't healthy, I hadn't yet figured out how to attain the right balance. That's another reason why I started Tammy Fit. Sharing recipes and meal plans and showing women that they should never starve themselves or eat boring, bland foods is really important. No-one should deprive themselves of one of life's greatest pleasures if they can help it.

If you stop and think about it for a moment, it's amazing to consider that with every mouthful you are choosing what to make yourself from. You are putting the building blocks of your body into your mouth. How your body develops depends, in part, on food. You literally build yourself each and every day! When you're making those decisions for your family too, it goes beyond choice. By teaching them what feels good and what tastes good, you're giving them a skill for life.

Of course, it can be tricky teaching kids about nutrition and good eating choices. It's important to let them have a few treats now and then. Sometimes I'll take the kids to the movies and let them have sweets, and we always celebrate with birthday cake, but for the most part, they really don't need sugary chemicals and trans fats whirling around their healthy little bodies. Keeping treats occasional keeps nutrition in balance; treats are a 'sometimes food', not an everyday one.

Although it can seem quicker and easier to buy fast food, cooking at home can be equally quick and simple. It's definitely healthier and usually tastes better too. Foods straight from nature are packed full of flavour and your body feels better after eating them. Think about how you feel after you eat something highly processed or full of fat – often heavy, bloated and a bit queasy. How do you feel after you eat something super sugary? Buzzing at first, but then sluggish and tired, right? Your body is talking to you. It's always talking to you, as I learnt from meditating. There's a reason you feel better when you eat fresh, wholesome, filling and delicious food. Your body craves it!

*

I fuel my body with whole, healthy food – lots of proteins, complex carbs and healthy fats. I also have a sweet tooth and love to treat myself occasionally with chocolate and ice cream. During the week I stick to lots of fruit and veg; protein in the form of chicken, tuna and yoghurt; and wholegrains such as rice and oats. On the weekends, I allow myself to indulge more, although I always balance it out with decent, healthy meals in between.

Some of my go-to meals are things like spaghetti bolognese, tuna sandwiches, chilli con carne, protein shakes or smoothies, or something as simple as a chicken stir-fry. When I feel like a snack, I'll grab some rice cakes with peanut butter and honey, or carrot sticks with hummus and chilli sauce. Or homemade zucchini fries! Yum. If you are making these things yourself from scratch and avoiding processed jars of sauces, it's quite easy to eat healthily.

A lot of people don't realise that some foods that are advertised as 'healthy' really aren't, for example, muesli bars or boxed cereals, both of which are packed full of sugar. So always read the labels! It's worth investing time into buying and preparing healthy food. It's what you and your loved ones are made of, after all.

Eat well

Diet and nutrition is a multi-billion-dollar industry, so I'm not here to break down the science behind it, just to give you the top-line healthy eating principles that work for me. It's not a diet or an eating plan or some complex theory you need a chemistry degree to comprehend, just a few simple steps to follow as a guide to a 'healthy eating life'. As a busy mum of three, eating this way keeps me energetic and feeling healthy and vital every day.

Ten steps for a 'healthy eating life'

1. Eat five smaller meals a day (forget the snacks).
2. Carbs are a good choice if you're exercising.
3. Make cooking fun and include your kids.
4. Add greens to pretty much everything.
5. Fuel up – eat for energy and strength.
6. Practise food gratitude – savour it.
7. If treats are occasional you'll enjoy them more.
8. Eat straight from nature whenever possible.
9. Listen to your body and how food feels.
10. Prep, prep, prep! The easier it is, the better.

When you
nourish your
body, you
nourish your soul.

MY FAVOURITE THING
(IS FOOD)

Aside from my family, food is one of my favourite things in the world. So is exercise. Living a full and busy life as mum to three young kids and running multiple businesses, plus my daily exercise, means I can eat well and eat a lot and stay fit and healthy. I have so many go-to meals and snacks that I love! My goal in this section is to give you a glimpse into what I put on my plate and what a typical eating day for me might look like . . . but before I do, a little word about what food can do for your mind and yes, even your soul.

When you nourish your body you feel good physically, but it also makes you feel good *mentally*. Not just for the pride in looking after yourself, but also the feel-good chemicals you're feeding your brain, such as the 'reward molecule' dopamine. For me, though, it's simpler than that. When you take the time to nurture yourself and your family, it's an act of love, a way of saying, 'I care about you'. I know first-hand how bad it feels not to care about your own wellbeing, so this is *incredibly* important. It's part of that big life goal, the thing you're showing up for most: happiness.

*

So, what to nourish yourself with? Here's an overview of my average day. Please know, however, it's important to modify any diet and exercise to suit your particular needs and lifestyle. Some of us are super active, while others are more sedentary – you'll need to adapt your food intake to suit that. The Tammy Fit app is filled with recipes, advice and ideas to support you on a daily basis if that's what you're looking for.

I'm someone who always has breakfast. I train early each day, so it makes sense for me to fuel my body for my workout. But even on my recovery days, I still eat first. Whether it's to fuel your mind or your body, I personally think breakfast is the most important meal of the day – it literally 'breaks your fast' from overnight, telling the body system to 'wake up' and get this day started. Until you fuel it, you will be on go-slow.

Across the day, carbs are something I welcome in my diet because I need them for energy. I try to get them mainly from plant-based, wholefood sources, avoiding things like boxed cereals and muesli bars, as they're full of sugar and add little nutritional value. At breakfast, oats are a particular favourite and I'll often add protein powder. Avocado and eggs on wholegrain toast is also a winner. Sneaking a bunch of greens into your shakes is a great way to increase fibre and antioxidants in your diet. I rarely eat bacon, sausages (or anything heavy or fatty), croissants or sweet breads, or juices which contain a lot of sugar.

After my workout I have protein powder in water, then mid-morning I eat a small meal of fresh fruit for healthy carbs – blueberries, bananas, watermelon, strawberries, grapes, pears and other fruits in season. I used to be stricter with eating too much fruit as it contains sugars, but these days I'm more flexible about that. Fruit can give you a sweet fix without all the nasty chemicals. It also contains a stack of other nutritional advantages which balances it out for me.

Lunch is often sandwich-based – an easy choice to have delivered or when eating out too. My sandwiches are full of lean

It's important for me to have high protein in every meal so I always add protein to my smoothies or breakfast bowls. ✨✨

protein and salad. Depending on how much energy I need, I may also add rice or sweet potato.

In the afternoons I'll have more of the same, or more fruit.

Dinner is my main meal with the family. I try to prep ahead, but if not, it's easy to put on some music and chop up lots of vegetables along with meat/seafood/chicken which I season, cook, then serve with rice, pasta or potatoes. I don't tend to eat anything after dinner, but I do love tea. I drink herbal teas – the naturally sweet-tasting ones help curb my sugar cravings.

On the weekends, I let my hair down and celebrate with parties and picnics with extended family and friends. We enjoy some drinks and stacks of seafood. There's always dessert or cheese platters and always lots of music. Food is glorious and part of nurturing yourself is knowing when to let go and celebrate. There are times to nurture yourself with routine and times when nurturing means throwing the rules out the window!

Food planning

You don't have to reinvent the wheel to make changes to your eating routine – often you just need to tweak things a little. Using the table over the page, review your regular eating habits to determine where you're choosing wisely and where you may need to improve.

MY FAVOURITE THING (IS FOOD)

I could do	Breakfast	Mid-morning	Lunch	Afternoon	Dinner	Weekends
More						
Less						

Don't get overwhelmed by overwhelm.

NOURISH
YOUR TIME

Now that we have nourishing your body sorted, let's look at how to nourish your mind. When it comes to nurturing your brain, stress is the enemy. 'Overwhelm' makes for a crappy life and it can creep up on you. One minute you feel like you're all over it, and the next you're over *everything*. Especially for mums or high achievers, it's too easy to crash into overwhelm, especially at certain busy times of the year. Suddenly your schedule is over full and you can't see how to clear space. Before you crash and burn, take a deep breath and look at your diary. Usually a few small tweaks to get rid of less important things and move other things around can buy you some breathing room. Because when it comes to overwhelm, you need to nourish your *time*.

*

It's hard to maintain a healthy life balance when you have too many balls in the air: kids, work, gym, social life, family. Most of us are juggling a lot already, so when a curve ball lobs in from left field, you're in serious danger of dropping the lot. It could be an argument, some bad news or a sudden worry; any added stress can quickly tip you into overwhelm.

Taking care of yourself and practising self-kindness will help ease the pressure; showing up for *you*. It can feel hard to do in the moment, when everyone's screaming at you to *get things done*, but sometimes taking an hour out is the only answer. The restorative calm will bring straight thinking and renewed energy and, more than likely, a boost of productivity. Yet so often we ignore the stress and think, 'I haven't got time for that right now'. Oh the irony. Time is *the point*. Thinking 'I'll be happy when this is done' is wasting a whole precious day of life – the chance to be happy *now*. Someone said to me once, 'Never dread the day ahead.' If you are? You're not *nourishing* time, you're *wasting* it.

I'm not talking about being 'busy' here. I love the excitement and buzz when things are happening and I'm getting stuff done. That's *good* busy. You want that. Overwhelm is different. Overwhelm is when you realise 'I *don't* want this'. That's *bad* busy.

When I get overwhelmed it's always preceded by signs that something is off – I get anxious or snappy, forgetful and unmotivated, even resentful. I know I've been guilty of pointing the finger, blaming a situation or, worse, someone else. *You made me feel this way!* But no-one can make you feel anything. Life is like a big mirror that you look into every day, choosing what you see and what you react to. People can give you *cause* to react but ultimately you must own it.

I find this concept liberating. *You can only control yourself, not anyone else.*

These days when overwhelm rears its unwelcome head, I take notice of what my body and mind are telling me – for example, headaches, feeling sluggish – and I don't delay. If you ignore the signs, chances are you'll fall in a heap and drop all your balls, usually at the most inconvenient time. I prefer to stay on the front foot, so when I see those wobbles appearing, I'm primed and ready to act.

The first thing I do is free up time by rearranging my meetings, centring them around certain days of the week. That way I can have a day or two to myself where I can schedule in some 'me time'. Fortunately, office work has allowed a lot of people more flexibility post-COVID, so hopefully this is something you can do too. Remember, your clients, boss, siblings, friends and family will take as much of you as you allow them to. It's up to you to change the set-up if it's not working for you. Better still, turn the tables! If you have kids, it might be time to call in the network – asking for help might only be a phone call away.

What I've learnt is that overwhelm is largely a time-management thing. So find a way to free some up. Better still, block in some 'me time' every week, now – *before* overwhelm has a chance to creep in. Life's too short and too beautiful to waste any of it feeling stressed and unhappy.

How overwhelmed are you?

Are you close to burnout? Let's find out. Consider everything you've done over the past two or three days and answer this:

- Have you been feeling down/snappy/not yourself?

- How many hours did you spend doing things you find fun?

- How many hours did you spend nurturing yourself?

If you are overwhelmed right now, I suggest you schedule in some of that 'good time' stuff. Only you really know where you're at – only you can take a hundred per cent care of yourself.

It's not you,
it's your DNA.

ALL OR NOTHING?

I want to delve a little more into this self-nurturing concept. It's clear I'm a fan of working hard to achieve my goals, but if I find myself continuously banging my head against a wall and not getting anywhere, I like to stop for a minute and recalibrate. *Is it time to tweak the process? What can I do to improve things?* Sometimes a small adjustment can make all the difference, but sometimes it needs more than that. Sometimes, as we discussed in the last chapter, what's required is to do *nothing*. And that's not me talking, that's our DNA.

*

At nineteen, pregnant and determined to build my own business, commitment became a lifeline for me. In *The Success Principles,* Jack Canfield says you have to be 'obsessed about success' and I took that on board. It was a healthy obsession which drove me forward in a positive way. With only $400 to my name, I needed blind faith and an almost fanatical commitment to my dream to give it any chance of success. I committed, gave it everything I had, and it worked. Because I'd put so much effort into building a strong foundation, later, when I needed to, I could pull back and bring others on board to help.

This is critical. Because no matter how committed you are, how strong you are, how willing you are, at some point, your body is going to ask you to slow down. We are not physically capable of going full tilt continuously without pause. Our bodies require downtime to absorb the changes that forceful effort delivers. The 'recovery period' is a critical part of a trainer's toolkit, because this is when adaptations occur. Without enough recovery, athletes can fall into an overtrained state. Depending on how deep they fall, it may take weeks or months to recover.

There's a scientific reason behind this; it's in our DNA. We've evolved biologically to react to stress with an adrenalin-based 'fight or flight' response. In today's world, we're more likely to be racing against a deadline than away from a deadly lion, but our nervous system doesn't know the difference. When we react to a threat – jungle predator, city traffic, or spreadsheet – our body releases adrenalin. Our bodies think they have to move *fast*. Our heart beats quicker, our breathing increases and blood flows rapidly from our core to our limbs. This is all great when you're trying to outrun that hungry lion, but in modern times, the fight or flight response makes us feel anxious and out of control.

A doctor friend of mine who lectures on this says that what we should do if we find ourselves in this state is: nothing. Well, practically nothing. Sleep, go for a little stroll, stare at the sky, meditate. Apparently doing 'nothing' triggers the opposite reaction to stress. It tells our bodies that everything is all right, that we don't need to run or hide or freak out. That all is well and here's some nice happy chemicals to prove it (endorphins, dopamine). It's in our DNA to stop and smell the roses – our bodies love it and reward us for it! And a lot of the time we need it more than we know.

'Nothing time' is valuable and can help manage anxiety. 'I'm just going to take a nana nap' isn't something to apologise for. Neither is, 'I spent the afternoon lazing about and

Allow yourself time to rest and just be.

staring into space.' You are doing something important for your health and it will make you feel better equipped to face challenges once you're all replenished and endorphined up. So if you feel you need it, take time out to do nothing. It's what you're programmed to do.

It's time to do . . . nothing

Do you spend much time doing nothing? If not, you should. Your body rewards you for relaxing. The right kind of rest will deliver performance gains. Get enough of it, and the good chemicals can eventually outweigh the stress-induced ones. Here's some do-almost-nothing activities I love. Feel free to add more of your own!

Sitting on a headland overlooking the ocean.

Lying on the grass finding pictures in the clouds.

Watching the sunset or sunrise.

Sitting in the forest and counting how many bird noises I can hear.

Wandering around looking into rock pools.

Studying a tree – every tiny detail.

Floating in the water.

Getting a massage.

Sitting in the hot tub.

Going to an art gallery and picking one piece to stare at.

Pottering in the garden and picking flowers.

Drifting along in a boat or taking a ferry.

Digging my toes in wet sand at the beach.

The ultimate
comeback is to
love your ~~way~~
self out of it.

THE POWER OF SELF-NURTURE

The trouble for most of us is that 'doing nothing' feels so useless. We're so conditioned to being busy and 'taking action' that when something huge happens, our first instinct is to make a move. But if you've just collided with disaster, your best move could actually be to stand still. It won't feel like it at the time, but situations like this can be some of the most powerful in your life, because you're going through spiritual growth.

We need adversity. We need challenge. At times it can feel almost impossible to get through. One of the hardest things you'll ever do is look for the light at the end of a very dark tunnel. When it feels as if the darkness will never lift, know this – no matter how long or how dark that tunnel, there *is* light at the end.

*

After my relationship break-ups, I was down. I mean, *really* hurting. Heartbreak stings and it takes time to get through the healing process, because part of that process is having to reinvent yourself, your life and your definition of family. It's grief, plain and simple. And grief is hard. Yet, it's an opportunity too, even though it can be difficult to see it that way.

Something has been lost, but that creates room to gain something new. The very first thing you need to gain is a new version of you. What do you look like now, on the inside? Who are you without that relationship? The ultimate comeback is to love yourself out of pain and emerge stronger and wiser than ever. Change can be hard, but it can also be good. Everything in life is temporary, remember? We're not meant to stay the same. The best thing you can do tomorrow is begin again.

But where do you start re-designing this new version of you? If you're a mum, your knee-jerk reaction is likely to look after everyone else first. But we've talked a lot about this – to be a good carer, you have to care for yourself first. It's not selfish, it's *necessary*. Your kids need this new version of you as much as you do! So start nurturing yourself. Practise self-care, don't put yourself second, and spend time doing things you enjoy to help you feel better.

It can be such a weird space at first, but by taking lots of positive small steps, you *will* figure this out. For me, doing things helped – exercising, meditating and reading. The beach and being in nature too. For you, it might be visiting friends, going to the movies, taking up painting. Doing things you love and trying new things you could learn to love will slowly but surely help you feel alive again. To like yourself again – maybe not the old self, but a new self. A better, stronger, wiser self.

People chase happiness like it's some kind of destination, but I think life's more about each and every day and evolving into a better place. You feel lost, then you find yourself again. Soul searching and healing may seem like life on pause, but in these moments you're taking a massive leap forward spiritually, so let it be what it is. There are no time limits – it will take as long as it takes. But over time, it *will* happen.

It's vital to know what you really want and, more importantly, how you want that to *feel*. I believe in manifestation and the laws of attraction, so I physically write down my goals, along with small, actionable steps. Then, little by little, I work towards them. They say the process of writing down your goals acts as a subconscious reinforcement, almost like a contract. You can also say them aloud to people you trust, as if making a promise. I used to set big money goals when I first started out, for example, intentions to make a certain amount in a year, but today my goals tend to be more emotion based, as in, 'I want to get up each day and feel really excited.' They're most powerful when stated in the present tense, as this shifts your belief system to act as if they're already true. So, for example, 'Every day I wake up feeling really excited again.'

This will help you reach the most important stage – gratitude. Fill yourself with gratitude for everything you are, everything you've achieved and everything you *will* achieve. That is the greatest manifestation of all.

Getting through tough times

Think about some of the hardest times of your life and what you did to get through. You may not realise it, but you probably already have some amazing tricks to help yourself get back on track. Sometimes it can be hard to remember them when you're in the tunnel, so here are some prompts to reflect upon:

1. What does courage look like for you? What have you done that was brave?

   ....

   ....

2. What was something that you thought you couldn't do, that you did? For example, starting a new job, moving overseas, finding a home.

   ....

   ....

3. What powerful sayings or songs have helped get you through tough times?

....

....

4. What positive 'I am . . .' statement can you write down, right now? For example, 'I am capable.'

....

....

Grateful for this body & all it does for me. For legs that can run, arms that can lift, lungs that can breathe. For the children it carried. Grateful to be able to train and do what I truly love. Grateful for my strength.

What you can
imagine, you
can have.

NOURISHING SELF-CONFIDENCE

Did you ever see that episode of *Seinfeld* when George reveals his secret about being a good liar? *If **you** believe it, it's true.* Self-confidence is a game you play with your mind. Whenever you tell yourself you *can't* do something, you start to believe it, and whenever you tell yourself you *can* do something, the same thing happens. Telling yourself constantly that you can, in fact *are already* doing something, is incredibly powerful. Nearly all those books in my step-dad's library talked about it. Visualising yourself at the top of your game is a form of mental programming – you're training your body to seek that feeling because it feels very, very good.

If you keep visualising your dream as your current reality, you're actively manifesting it into being, because your focus is always directed towards that goal. By taking the dream seriously, you're making a commitment to it. Every time you envisage it and imagine how success feels, you are improving your chances of attaining it. This tool is so valuable that professional athletes spend a lot of time and money working with sports psychologists to visualise their future success. Belief = confidence = reality. Taking real-life, practical steps towards your goal is important too, but if you consistently practise your skills and visualise your

I honestly never thought my core would be as strong after having 3 kids. Core work used to be SO daunting to me & I'd try to avoid it wherever I could. I can honestly say, little by little, I've built back the strength & MORE (which I'm very proud of 😌). It's definitely NOT about the aesthetics.

success, you're building both physical *and* mental pathways. Don't just do it once and think 'I'm done'. What you can imagine, you can have, but it requires constant practice to get there.

*

When I first started out, I thought achievement was all about *doing* things. Going to the gym, eating well, showing up. But the more my ambition grew, the more I realised that achievement was equally a mental game. The more I focused on getting *where* I wanted to be, the quicker I got there.

It's hard to remain fully focused on your big dream sometimes, yet focus is the key. If you can program yourself into having a strong, positive attitude towards something, it will come to pass. Self-belief drives the sass that's so powerful it can feel like magic. As if you're invincible! Really, you're confident.

As with anything, building your self-confidence requires nourishment. Demonstrate your belief by regularly writing your dreams down and saying them out loud. Make them *specific*. Say them often. Create a step-by-step plan and accomplish a small goal each day. Remember, you are following your heart's desire. Reward your achievements along the way and before you know it, you'll have reached your goal.

1. **Set goals.** I don't take goal-setting lightly, not because I'm worried I might not achieve it – because I believe I will! I don't set goals once in a blue moon, either. Life changes, so the goal posts regularly need resetting. The clearer you are, the better.

2. **Write them down and say them out loud.** If you can imagine it, you can have it, so imagine your dream being true in as much detail as possible. Putting pictures on your fridge or screen saver can act as great visual reminders. Regularly say your goals out loud – to your inner circle, or even to the mirror.

3. **Make a step-by-step plan.** I write each step, right from the present moment, all the way up to achieving my dream, getting very specific and making a clear schedule. Then? I stick to it! Every time I tick something off I get a sweet little buzz of achievement. Sometimes I give myself a real reward too – spa days are nice.

Set yourself a goal

Is there something you want to achieve, yet you're struggling with self-confidence and self-belief? Time to write down that goal (very specifically), say it out loud and make a clear plan.

My very specific goal:

....

....

....

My step-by-step plan:

....

....

....

Prompts I'll use to inspire and remind me:

....

....

....

Count the
blessings money
can't buy.

IT'S ALL
ABOUT LOVE

Can you really have it all? Well, that depends on what you think 'it all' is. Some people think making a success of yourself revolves entirely around money and career achievement, but that isn't true. I love the saying, 'Always count the blessings money can't buy.' It isn't what you physically have that matters – someone can be super rich and famous, yet wandering around their big old house alone, feeling depressed. Another person could be living simply but feel happy, surrounded by love, laughter and family.

It's all about perspective. Mostly, it's all about love. To round out this section on nourishment, I want to finish off with an important message: nothing nourishes like love. It's the only thing that really matters when it all comes down to it.

*

Throughout my life I've been poor, lived in a mansion, struggled, then become wealthy again. My financial circumstances have changed a lot, but did they truly affect my happiness? I'm often asked, 'Don't you feel guilty for having money? How shallow and materialistic are you now?'

Honestly, I don't think I am. Shallow people don't see the depth in life: in others, the things around them, the moments that matter. If anything, I see depth in *everything*. So calling me shallow? I don't think that's fair. If anything, I'm possibly *too* deep and emotional, but I'm okay with that.

And materialistic? I wouldn't say yes to that, either. From all I've experienced, I am now so grateful for the wealth I've managed to create and I love the lifestyle my efforts afford me. Do I take it for granted? No. Do I appreciate it? Every day. Do I feel the need to apologise for it? I don't. I work hard every day and continue to create opportunities for others. Actually, I'm proud of the money I make.

Achieving wealth and success was just *one* part of my big dream. I know plenty of people who've worked just as hard as me and that I've been very lucky the way things have panned out. Some of my experiences have been surreal, like flying on a private jet from LA to New York for our first Saski NYFW show. Still, they were *moments* rather than material things. Experiences only money can buy, sure, but alongside that unmatchable high of achieving a hard-won goal, the people I was sharing them with was what made those experiences special.

For me, the biggest moments in life are all about love and connection. The highs are so much higher when you have someone to enjoy them with. There's an age-old question: if a tree falls in a forest, but no-one sees it, did it ever fall? I can fly overnight to LA by myself, but if there's someone there to giggle with en route, it's so much better. To put it in perspective, no jet plane ride to a cool destination could even *remotely* compare to the moments when my three babies were born. Life is about moments – big and small – and the connections they create.

A big fancy house and a nice car are just *things*. It's the people *inside* a house that make it a home, the little cherubs in the safety seats that matter. The rewards of money are the memories I've been able to make with my loved ones. Travels and adventures, dinners and shopping. More importantly, being able to help out family members and set up my kids for the future. The most

To raise you gently & selflessly. To never let you doubt for a second how important you are. To love you deeply with a love that transcends all else. To protect you fiercely. To guide you with kindness & understanding.

fun we have is watching movies together and chasing each other along the beach. You don't need money to have fun. Underneath my high-profile job, I'm still just a regular person. Deep down, the core of me is the same. I make mistakes, I struggle and I'm constantly learning.

No matter how 'successful' you are, I believe you should continue on the path of personal growth and self-development. For me that hasn't changed. When asked if I feel guilty about money and success, I have to say no, I don't. Because I've discovered that, in the end, the real happiness lies in sharing it all and I definitely *don't* feel guilty about that. I just feel grateful.

Money and success are not the be all and end all. Love is. That's the true wealth. Spending time with the people I care about, nourishing them and our relationship, and nurturing what I do and who I do it with are my true blessings in life. To me that's really 'having it all'.

Having it all
How much of 'it all' do you have? More than you realise. It's time to count your blessings.

I am blessed because I have:

....

....

....

I am blessed because I feel:

....

....

....

PARENTING

As you know by now, my family is the centre of my world. My kids are everything to me and I am super close with my siblings, nieces and nephews. For me, prioritising family is so important because they're my confidants, colleagues and friends too. I want my children to grow up feeling the massive love of family and knowing I gave them my time and attention. I want them to know they're loved unconditionally.

Among the lifestyle changes that came with moving between Queensland and Singapore, one of the biggest was becoming part of an extended family. It wasn't just Mum, Dad, Emilee, Amy and me anymore. My mum had all three of us girls really young, by twenty-three. When she met my step-dad she went on to have several more children. So I am one of seven siblings. Being part of such a large family has taught me a lot, some of which I'll share with you here.

In the TV show *Modern Family*, older dad Jay and his second wife Gloria have a somewhat complicated relationship with their kids from different partners. Jay's are adults with kids of their own, while Gloria's son Manny is still in school. Gloria's ex keeps letting Manny down – not picking him up and doing his dad weekends. When, yet again, he fails to take Manny on a promised trip to Disneyland, Jay takes him instead. 'There's no real secret to being a good parent,' Jay says. 'It's often just showing up.'

As with everything else in this book, showing up for your family is *everything*. It's not just words; it's being there, both *physically* and *emotionally*. It's showing commitment. Demonstrating how much you care. Giving your kids your time is showing up for love. And that's not only a gift for childhood, it's a gift for life.

Happy Mother's Day to all the mamas! To the single mamas playing both roles, to those with mamas in heaven & to the ones yearning to be mamas. Thinking of you today & every day.

To my little ones, thank you for giving me the best job in the world.
For showing me a love I never knew possible.
For teaching me so much.
For helping me realise my own strength & for growing alongside me everyday.

So beyond grateful. 🫶

Happiness is always the best choice to make, long term.

MODERN HAPPY FAMILIES

My parents got divorced when I was young, then as an adult I split up with both my kids' dads. Separation or divorce are the last things anyone wants to happen once you have a child together – to have to raise them separately – but I've come to learn that it's far better to reinvent than remain stuck in a cycle of unhappiness. Break-ups are incredibly painful to go through, but it's better than spending years, maybe your whole life, in pain.

Deciding to leave my kids' dads was incredibly painful. You feel guilty for repeating the same cycle, having sworn it would never be you. You start to second-guess all your decisions.

On the flipside, you also know from experience that there's life beyond divorce – good life, too. Modern happy families are often *extended* happy families. If the alternative to splitting up is for everyone to remain miserable, it's far better to split. Happiness is always the best choice to make, long term, but only you can decide what that means for you. For me, I could only take into account what we were experiencing and what I knew from my own childhood. In the end, separating was the only real choice.

*

Being 1 of 7 has always been
one of my greatest blessings.
one of my greatest blessings.
My siblings are my whole life. ♡♡
My newest baby girl doesn't realise
how blessed she is. Already has
2 best friends & lifelong protectors.
 🔒

We can learn so much from our own upbringing – good and bad – and what we want to bring to the table when it's our turn to raise little humans. Being the child of divorce has so many implications. Your parents try as hard as they can to protect you, but kids see and hear much more than adults think. Emilee and Amy remember a lot more than me because I was the youngest, but I do have flashbacks of feeling really sad that Mum and Dad were arguing all the time. Still, they were clearly not meant to stay together. Looking at them now, even the idea of it has us shaking our heads. They are way too different.

Between my mum, my sisters and my dad, I was very protected from the drama of the divorce – being the youngest, they always looked out for me. Nonetheless, I learnt some big life lessons from it all, and overcame a lot of fears. Since my own separations, I've got experience from the other side too. Here are some things that helped me get through:

1. Just because your parents don't want to be a couple anymore, it doesn't mean they don't love you.
2. Your step-parent won't necessarily be like the evil step-mum in *Cinderella* – they could love you like their own child.
3. The modern family model of being an extended family can end up being more people for you to love.
4. It takes a village to raise a child, in my case, a family village.
5. Family can take many forms and relationships can too.
6. It doesn't matter where you are, it's who loves you that matters. Home is always where the heart is.

Ultimately, all three of my parents have had a huge, positive impact on my life. I feel incredibly blessed about that because I know a lot of people don't have the same experience – whether from an extended family or not. Whatever your upbringing has been like, I hope you can embrace the positives and somehow let go of any old hurts. The more you can do that, the better it will be for your kids, and for you. But don't be too hard on yourself and that child inside. Get help if you need it, be open to healing. And be gentle with yourself, okay?

Parental advice

Thinking back to when you were a child, what advice would you give to yourself about being a parent now? Are you giving yourself some love and appreciation for all the things you're doing right? It's so important. Gratitude towards yourself matters so much when you're a parent. Here are two things to reflect on:

The advice I would give from childhood me:

....

....

....

Some love and appreciation to myself for what I'm doing right:

....

....

....

If it's a priority,
there's always
time.

MAKE TIME

Time is the excuse, or the reason we all give for not showing up. It's funny when you think about how we try to explain it away, as if we just 'ran out of it', or 'couldn't find it' or weren't 'able to make the time'. We hold our hands up in the air and say, 'Where did it go?' as if there's some cosmic magic trick going on. Here's the thing about time, though: *it's finite*. There are only so many hours in the day and the good part about that is you can *plan*. Time doesn't have to be this mysterious substance that goes missing, it's right here. There *are* enough hours in the day and we *have* got time for that – if 'that' is a priority.

Showing up as a parent requires plenty of time, no denying. What hours you choose to make *your* time or someone else's is the bigger question.

*

When my kids and businesses were infants, I really struggled with this issue. I became completely overwhelmed trying to spend time with the kids *and* on work *and* on everything else all at once. Asking for help is important, but knowing *what* to ask for can be tricky. What should you outsource and what should you keep for yourself?

Being a hands-on mum is something I love and although it can be hard sometimes, I remind myself that my kids won't be this little forever. I strive to be as involved as I possibly can. On the other hand . . . everything and everyone else needs my time too. So I've become much better at prioritising.

Certain things are *mine* and non-negotiable. School drop-offs are one, and if the kids are getting up in front of the school or performing or something, there's no way I'm missing that either. I couldn't stand to think of their little faces searching the crowd, hoping I was there and I wasn't. If it's their priority, then it's mine. After all, I won't remember the deadline that got pushed, but they'll sure remember how I showed up for them.

I think the primary school years are easier when it comes to time management because your days are very structured. The baby and preschool years are a bit more all over the place because your kids are so dependent on you. Some days you have to drop everything for them. I often felt paranoid when they were really small. When each of my kids was born I was terrified of *anything* happening to them. The world felt filled with dangers. That was another part of the reason I became so overwhelmed – I was trying to protect them all by myself from *everything*.

Po is still a baby as I'm writing this book, so I am currently taking her into the office with me which suits us both and is so hilarious. Mayhem, but hilarious. It definitely isn't easy trying to get work done when she's climbing all over the keyboard or hiding behind the screen in meetings but, between my work family and me, we've figured out ways to manage. I've set up a play pen in the office and I bring in plenty of toys and snacks so she is occupied (sort of). I know how precious this time is and how quickly it will go, so I'm trying to make the absolute most of it.

For me, another non-negotiable 'mum time' is before and after work. Kids need routine and I want to be there to give them that. Our morning routine consists of breakfast and

A whole two months since I gave life to my third little being & feeling so good. Slowly restoring my core strength. A long way to go in my overall strength but I'm enjoying the ride & taking my time. Training is my happy place, my me time, my mental sanctuary & I'm coming back stronger than everrr – watch this space!

getting ready (+ general chaos) and after school I usually cook everyone dinner while the kids do their reading, homework, music practice (+ general chaos) before it's time for baths, then TV time in Mummy's room. I love this part of the day. It's just us. I find it the most precious use of time imaginable, tucking them in and singing 'You Are My Sunshine'.

My dad always sang that song to my sisters and me, and I have sung it to my kids ever since they were babies. It's part of our little bedtime ritual. Seeing how happy it makes them warms my heart. Dad still sings it to me and I don't think I'll ever stop singing it to my kids. It ties his love into our home. The best thing about bringing your childhood with you, is that it brings your parents along with you too.

Precious moments

Name some precious moments in your routine. What would you like to do more of and what could you give away that isn't a priority?

How I'm spending my time	Am I happy with the time I spend on it?	Ways to increase or decrease this accordingly

How I'm spending my time	Am I happy with the time I spend on it?	Ways to increase or decrease this accordingly

All the small
things add up
to big love.

PRIORITIES

Mother Teresa believed, 'We can do no great things, only small things with great love.' I think this is most true when applied to kids. Making sandcastles. Playing dress-ups. Reading stories. You can buy your baby a tricycle, but she'll want to play with the box.

Maybe because of my carefree childhood in the rainforest, my family loves being outdoors. We all love music, parties and food. Hugs and laughter. Dancing. Small things and simple things. They really are the best.

*

After a hard week's work, I always plan a fun activity to do together on weekends. Since being in nature was such a big part of my own childhood, I like to get the family outdoors. We go to the beach or park or have a nice picnic somewhere and invite all the cousins. We also love movie nights at home with the full set-up: big screen, popcorn and blankets. Doing fun things together doesn't take much, just time and imagination.

Everyday routines matter too. Simple tasks done well. Kids thrive on routines because they send the message that all is safe and well – they find comfort in their familiarity. And every parent knows the feeling of accomplishment that comes from getting everyone fed and bathed for the night. I make it a priority to take the kids through their evening routine. Often that means I'll be back online after they're in bed, but it's worth it.

As the business decision-maker, I have to be on my phone constantly for work. Managing this is probably one of my hardest challenges because I have to divide my attention. I can often manage to have one ear out for work and another for the kids, but sometimes I just have to turn the phone off and be there for my munchkins. Mother's intuition tells me when.

There are plenty of days when the laundry's piled up, the house is a mess and the kids are calling for me. Meanwhile, I have deadlines to meet and people pulling me in ten different directions. When I find myself in the middle of such a storm I know I must stop and obey the golden rule of success: do the most important thing first. Depending on time constraints, people's emotional needs, or client demands, that could be anything from making a fashion-line decision for work, or listening to Wolf practise his speech for school.

How do I know which to choose? I trust my instincts. Also, if it can be done in ten minutes or less, it's worth crossing off my to-do list. Not only does that shorten my list but it's amazing how much mental space I get back once I cross something off. Each small achievement contributes to the bigger picture, so by nailing one thing, then the next, I make progress. Even if I don't achieve everything, the important things get done. Laundry can always wait. Unless it's sports day tomorrow!

Focus on the small things

It's worth pausing to reflect on what makes you happy. Often it's the smallest things, in which case it won't take much to bring you back to your regular routine.

- What little things do you remember from childhood that meant a lot to you?

....

....

....

- What little things could you bring into your life now that would make a big difference?

....

....

....

You'll always
be a work in
progress.

HANDS UP WHO
<3 THEMSELVES

I've come to realise that you are and always will be a work in progress. Some days, the best version of you is standing in front of the mirror, wearing a new outfit, with your hair and make-up done, reflecting on how well you did being a mum today and smashing goals at work. Other days, the best version of you might be curled up in bed, binge-watching Netflix and eating ice-cream because today sucked and you need some self-care.

The 'best' you is always relative to where you're at right now. Accepting that is part of building a better you. Our overarching commitment is to be the *best version* of ourselves, which some-times means taking the pressure off. Work, friends, romance, parenting? It's a lot. Be your own cheer squad and make sure you're not letting any negative self-talk bring you undone. Life's hard enough.

Motherhood has taught me to be kinder to myself because in your kids' eyes, you're the sun and the moon. They see the world so innocently and generously. Saskia is the kindest person and Wolf is everyone's little champion. If only adults could view things with the pure hearts of kids! They have definitely reframed my priorities and outlook.

*

I was twenty when I had Wolf. That's when I think my self-growth and success journey really began. I've been on that path ever since and the challenges have helped me become a better person. Funny, isn't it, how people said motherhood would 'ruin everything'? For me, the *opposite* was true.

Motherhood forced me to grow up and move into a new stage of life. It brought an all-consuming love which almost burnt me until I learnt to look after myself too. My kids have taught me not to take life too seriously. They've taught me how to have fun. Sometimes it feels like the work will never end, and then *boom*! Wolf's at school. Where has the time gone?

I've learnt the importance of slowing down and appreciating where you're at. Too often people are in a rush to get somewhere, striving to achieve all these goals without enjoying the process. They don't stop and smell the roses. They lose sight of the little, precious things right in front of their noses. They don't value the moment they're in. I know, because I've done it!

The best way to get the most from life is to *savour* it. Slow down and appreciate what you're going through. It's easy to get down on yourself if you're not making the progress you want. But tomorrow never comes and the past is already over. Honestly, you only have *right now*. So what are you going to do with it?

I was thinking about internal dialogues recently, about all those things we say to ourselves, good and bad. I talk to myself constantly, both in my head and aloud. Back in my late teens I had some serious negative self-talk going on. Now it's very different – I'm back as I was, age twelve. I used to talk to myself in the mirror a lot then. I'd say to my reflection, 'You've got this, girl.' Looking at myself in the mirror nowadays I see someone who tries every day, someone who's striving to be the best version of herself, the woman who's raising my kids. She deserves love, that woman, because she is all that I am.

There is no darkness that
cannot be overcome by light.
Keep shining.

Self-reflection

How kind and supportive are you towards yourself? Or are you being overly self-critical? It's worth becoming aware of your internal dialogue and flipping the script if you need to. Next time you catch yourself saying something negative, redirect it with a positive.

Negative self-talk is so common, you might recognise the statements below. Add your own scripts to the list, find a way to counter them, then start applying positive redirection.

Negative	Positive
You are so disorganised and hopeless.	You're so creative. Let's harness it using a better system, shall we?
Why are you always so late?	It's great that you love not wasting a minute, but if you arrive early, you'll have time to catch up on emails and social feeds.
Why are you eating that? You have no self-control.	Eat slowly and enjoy every last bite. We can make healthier choices tomorrow.

Negative	Positive

Get rid of
the guilt, sit
back . . . and
smile.

MUM GUILT

Ah, mum guilt. Even though you know your work–life balance will never be perfect, guilt still comes with the territory, especially for career mums. Worse, I have guilt about mum guilt because I know I shouldn't feel it! But we all do. Like many parents, I have very high expectations of myself, but I've learnt that I'm never going to be perfect and I don't have to be.

Mind you, I still have those moments when the guilt creeps back in, the FOMO too. I might miss out on an assembly, or forget about crazy sock day, and I find myself wishing I could be that full-on mum who goes to *all* the meetings and activities and *never* misses a thing. But I *can't* be that and have everything else in my life ticking along too. The reality is that I *do* have to run the businesses, I *do* have to go to the gym to make this all work, and I *am* responsible for other people's livelihoods.

It's such a shame that working mums have to wrangle with these feelings of not being enough for our kids who we love so much. There are so many positives that we could be focusing on instead; wonderful qualities that you develop as a parent. For my part, I know I have patience now that I certainly never had before and a depth of love and protectiveness that only having a child can teach you. Most of us grow as compassionate human beings once we become mums and are doing an incredible job of loving and nurturing our children – yet we are the *last* ones to tell ourselves that. Mums and dads and other carers too are often harder on themselves than anyone else.

I've had to really work on the mum guilt stuff, something made even harder with trolls judging my every move, but I believe in showing my son and daughters that a woman can be whatever she wants to be and *still* be a good mum. She can be a strong leader, build something that benefits many, and can entertain, motivate and inspire on a massive scale.

Mum can be healthy and fit and strong and she can make that a priority. She can also give her kids opportunities to see and experience wonderful things around the world while still being there for them when they come home to everyday homework and swimming lessons. Everything I do centres around being a well-rounded person and a strong woman. But most of all, being a good mum. That's my goal, every day, and it's why I do what I do.

I'm a work in progress, as all mums are, and every night I sit back, take stock and ask myself if there are ways I could improve tomorrow. Of course I can, because I'm not perfect. Sometimes I lose my patience and get mad, or forget to do something, or don't pay attention to what they're saying. It's so easy to be hard on yourself, but the funny thing is, it's *just as easy* to be kind to yourself.

Once I decide on the things I want to improve, I reflect on the things I'm doing well. And yes, this is hard too! There's no job on earth that is going to make you more self-critical than parenting, but trust me, you *are* doing great things. You made them feel special with that little note in their lunchbox, you had them in stitches when you sang that Taylor Swift song (badly) in the car, you noticed that one of them felt a bit left out at the park and needed a hug. You did all of those things. Acknowledge yourself and hold onto those precious moments. Get rid of the guilt, sit back . . . and smile.

No more mum guilt!

1. What wonderful things has being a mum/dad/carer taught me?

....

....

....

2. These are the ways I'd like to do a bit better:

....

....

....

3. These are the ways I know I'm doing a great job:

....

....

....

4. Being a mum/dad/carer makes me grateful because:

....

....

....

Nurture their
nature.

LITTLE MIRRORS

I find it fascinating that when you meet a baby for the very first time, you're also meeting the adult they will one day become. We are all born with an innate personality, with certain traits, qualities and dispositions. It's bittersweet seeing your babies develop as they progress through all their stages. One minute they're a part of you, next they're permanently attached to you, and then *boom*! Suddenly they're walking. They go from newborn, to eating food, holding a bottle, laughing, crawling, to eventually walking and saying your name! All in the blink of an eye. It's just mind-blowing when you think about it.

Throughout it all, they will do it their way, in their style, following their mood. This presents its own challenges. When kids are being their stubborn selves, it's easy to lose patience. The secret is to work *with* their nature, not *against* it – to teach them how to make it work to their advantage.

*

Sometimes your kids are so much like you it's spooky. Saskia is such an active sleeper, just like me. I've always been restless in bed; I kick and toss and turn. She's the same. If we're not careful, we can end up in a boxing match while fast asleep – we don't even know we're doing it! We roll around so much, we're likely to fall out of bed.

They also share some of my other personality traits. Do we call it stubborn or determined? Shy or thoughtful? Dreamy or creative? It's easy to apply negative labels, but be careful. Your kids are little sponges and will believe *everything* you tell them. My job as a parent is to be their personal cheer squad. I want to fill their heads with positive self-talk so I'm always talking them up, telling them how great they are, how imaginative, energetic and creative. What you believe, you will become, and I want my kids to believe they are capable of achieving *anything*. That's certainly what my parents taught me.

All you ever want for your kids is to be happy. Happy babies, happy kids, happy teens, happy adults. As a parent, that can be tricky. For example, when do you push and when do you allow them to just float? My take on that is to be gentle. I don't believe in heaping expectation on their shoulders, rather, uplifting and encouraging them to believe in themselves.

Sometimes that comes down to discipline. Once again, I try to do this gently while at the same time being firm. Kids will test your patience. It can feel so much easier to give in – we all do sometimes. But do it all the time and they will start seeing you as a pushover and take advantage of it. *Kids need boundaries.* These should be held consistently by all their main carers so they don't get mixed messages. One line, held firm. There's safety in that.

If Mum says 'no', but Grandma says 'yes', it's confusing. Smart kids will learn to manipulate those situations to their advantage and I don't think that's the right lesson to be teaching them. Fortunately, my kids' dads and I are on the same page with this.

It's the same when they throw a tantrum, especially out in public. They may be small, but these little humans are talented guilt trippers. They're not trying to be malicious, they're just figuring out how the world works. If you let them win by

Our children are our mirrors.
Be kind to yourself and others.

manipulating you, that's the wrong character trait to be developing. While you'll be sorely tempted to give in to their red-faced demands in the lolly section of Coles, rewarding bad behaviour never ends well in the long run.

Ultimately, they will learn how to behave from watching you. You are constantly setting the example. If you lose it, they're watching. If you cry, they're watching. If you're calm and composed, they're watching. As I say, kids are little sponges. How about when they mimic things you say, like, 'That's the best thing *ever!*' – cute. Or, 'I am sooo over this!' – oops.

They are little mirrors, but one of my older friends told me a story that gives me hope. She asked her twenty-year-old son if he thought she and her partner had done a good job raising him. 'Of course you did,' he said. 'Look at me – I'm *awesome!*' Humblebrag aside, he genuinely *is* awesome. I hope one day my little tribe says the same about themselves – and me.

Bring out the best in them

Are your kids like you in certain ways? Do they have other traits that can be both positive and negative? Have a think about what they are and what you can do to best nurture their nature:

Trait	How to best nurture that trait

Trait	How to best nurture that trait

You are
endlessly
capable.

UNDERLYING VALUES

When it comes to being the best parent you possibly can be, let your values be your roadmap. Perhaps you've never really thought about them, yet they are *seriously* important. Values underscore every single thing you do whether you're aware of them or not. They're more than morals, they're *belief systems*. Experts say they are instilled in you from a very young age and show up at crucial points in your life. This was certainly true for me – once I saw my how my values and belief system affected my behaviour, everything made so much more sense.

*

My relationship values developed when I was very young. I think they do for everyone, but none more obviously than in a child of divorced parents. I learnt that the modern family model *can* work, and also, that kids see more than you think.

Because of that, I never wanted my kids to witness any problems between their parents. One thing I was determined *never* to do was to say a bad word about their fathers, either in front of them or in public. They don't want to hear it and they don't need to. I've tried my absolute best to stick to that and to set a good example for them as they start to develop their own relationship values.

I'm not saying it was easy. It was hard. It's difficult to control your emotions and put on a brave face when you're desperately trying to hide your pain and frustration. It's tempting to argue and strike out because you *are* hurt, you *are* angry, but that accomplishes nothing. Everyone has their own perceptions and feelings, so when things are difficult you just need to focus on your behaviour. What can *you* do to make the situation better? You can't control the other person, but you *can* control yourself.

I'm so grateful for the strength motherhood has given me to get me through those times, and I'm glad to say I'm in a good place with the kids' dads now. My parents and step-dad taught me that life after break-ups can work, and to be in an extended, loving family is *awesome*. No model of family is better or worse than another. Love is love and if you're surrounded by it every day, you're blessed.

Aside from my kids, the relationships I have with my immediate family are the most important in my world. We are incredibly close and no-one else will ever have those shared experiences. No-one else will ever know, understand and love you like your parents and siblings. To me, that is sacred. My family taught me my earliest lessons in life and they still guide everything I do. They formed my first values and they are my first priority.

All the moving around and facing new challenges, and being one of seven and living out of suitcases on big trips or running wild in the forest . . . all of it taught me how to be me. It gave me resilience and strength. My family has my back, and I have theirs. No matter what.

So when it comes to passing onto my kids what my parents valued most – what I now value too – it's those three invaluable principles: value your family, value working things out, and value your inner strength. After all, you are *endlessly* capable. I want my children to believe that about themselves more than anything, every single day.

Values and belief system

What values underpin your belief system and subconsciously influence everything you do? If you're not sure, it can help to think of some extreme situations or big decisions you've faced. How did you respond? What values drove that behaviour?

Big life decisions or circumstances	Your response – what action did you take?	What beliefs or values drove that behaviour?

Brought in the new year the only
way I'd want to – relaxing at home
with my little loves. Grateful for
the year that was. The year that
taught me I can quite literally
handle anything. The year I met
my little Posy worm. The year
I learnt the most about myself,
more than ever before. Bring
on more years of growth, love &
happiness. Wishing nothing but
love & success for every single
one of you. 📖

CHALLENGES

You don't get through life without facing challenges; they're just part of the deal. Do I love them? Probably not at the time. Do I value them? Wholeheartedly. Challenges build character – without them we'd be going nowhere fast. From the minute I decided to launch my own business, the challenges came marching in.

There I was with two little kids, a booming app, a successful fashion line, and it all kept growing and growing. Soon I was able to open office spaces and warehouses for both businesses, and hire employees, which was such a great feeling. Surreal but great. If my relationship hadn't been falling apart it would have been perfect. Although I was mostly figuring things out as we went along, it was fun and I was super confident I was going to be successful. At times though, all that pressure felt enormous.

Backing yourself isn't always easy. It's interesting to see how different people handle it. Some give up at the first hurdle. Some get their fingers burnt and become timid but willing to try again on a smaller scale. Others respond to a setback with all guns blazing, more determined than ever to succeed. Challenges can be a bit like a game of Truth or Dare. It reveals a person's true strength and just how daring they're willing to be.

This goes beyond business. To pick yourself up from emotional rock bottom takes more courage than anything. No challenge will ever test you more than that. In response you'll need determination, positivity, resilience and a *very* thick skin. But most of all, you'll need a big reason to drag yourself out of the depths of despair and come back stronger than ever. That reason is, almost always, love.

View mistakes not as something negative, but as an opportunity to improve.

If it doesn't feel right, it probably isn't. If it _does_ feel right, it probably is.

GO WITH YOUR GUT

I am a big believer in going with your gut. Deep down I think you *always* know what the answer is, but it gets clouded along the way. Other people's opinions muddy the waters. Flattery and promises put stars in your eyes.

If you get overexcited about what you're doing, there's a danger you might not think things through properly. Guilty! Jumping in head first can be both good and bad. It's true that overthinking can get in the way and that action delivers results. But if you act *too* fast and mistakes get made, you'll have plenty of time to live in regret.

*

The early days of launching Saski were a whirlwind. Everything was happening so fast that most decisions were made on the fly. Mine, anyway. Amy was far more organised. Her attention to detail and level head made her the perfect partner at the time. She balanced out my total lack of fear and spontaneity.

Ready for launch, we'd pulled together an impressive clothing line and were confident the orders would pile in. We pressed 'go', and . . . right from the start, disaster struck. Somehow the website allowed the overselling of a product we had no stock of!

We received *hundreds* of orders that couldn't be fulfilled. *Ding, ding, ding.* The orders kept piling in. We were running about the room, freaking out and screaming, 'What do we do?!'

After we'd finally managed to shut down the order process, we still had hundreds of customers to deal with. It seemed the only answer was to send an email explaining the mistake and offering to refund their money. But I had worked in customer service, remember? Although I'd hated that call centre job, I'd also learnt how to deal with people. I knew an impersonal message would not cut it, especially with my brand at its centre. People would feel that I had *personally* let them down, and I couldn't bear that.

Maybe it didn't really matter, but the first impression those customers formed of Saski mattered a *lot* to me. My instinct was telling me that emailing them was the wrong move and when my intuition is ringing alarm bells, I listen. 'The phone is king,' my gut was whispering – an old line from my telemarketing days. Isn't it funny how something that seemed such a total waste of time can return when you least expect it, delivering something of value after all?

I knew that phoning our customers would take time, so we sent the emails too. Yet I also rang each and every one of those customers personally to apologise, and they were so incredibly nice. A few really seemed to appreciate chatting to me in person too. In some ways, it made the whole thing a pleasant experience. Finally, with the disaster behind us and despite its terrible start, my second business became another big hit.

I learnt something important about business that day: always treat every customer like they're your *only* customer and you can't go wrong. That ideal has evolved over the years to: always treat every *person* like they're the only person who matters in that moment and you can't go wrong. In business, in my personal life, among my family and friends, I try to be fully present when I am with someone. It makes the experience so much richer.

Perhaps more importantly, the orders debacle reiterated to me how important it is to check in with yourself. My intuition saved us that day. In this noisy world, it's hard to hear properly sometimes. You must get quiet to go within. Trust me, listening to those whispers will change your world. The strongest message my gut tells me is to back myself. Trust myself. You have the answers inside you.

Listen to your intuition

Are you wrestling with a decision and finding it hard to decide what to do? Answering these questions should help you communicate with your intuition.

What you are trying to decide – write it down:

....

What are the pros?

....

What are the cons?

....

Now that you've considered it logically, let's apply some emotion. How would you advise someone you love to proceed?

....

Remember, gut = intuition = trusting yourself.

Trust is easy
until it's broken.
After that it's
hard.

LITTLE FISH,
BIG OCEAN

In the early days of parenting my first two babies and my first two businesses, things were coming at me thick and fast. Over-whelm reared its ugly head and, looking back, I can see that the choices I made would likely never have happened if I hadn't been running around a million miles an hour, trying to do everything and be everything to everyone. But back then, all I could see were my commitments, responsibilities and the push to build an even bigger dream. There wasn't enough time to think beyond what seemed most important: the break-up, my kids and making these businesses successful. The external noises were so loud, I stopped hearing my internal voice. Instead of trusting my gut instinct, I began trusting the wrong people and looking in the wrong places.

*

By my early twenties, my businesses were expanding fast. Oppor-tunity was knocking and timing is everything. I knew I had to capitalise on the success of Tammy Fit and Saski. My brands had global reach. To take them to the next level, I had to conquer the US. I was motivated and had the belief, but big business doesn't come with a guidebook. Arriving to the LA business scene,

It's not real over there. I was chasing something that I thought was all glitz and glam – a lifestyle that I wanted. And then I slowly realised that a lot of the people I met and the people I knew were just very toxic, not nice people at all. It was all very materialistic and ultimately not what I really thought life was about.

I found myself in unfamiliar territory – I didn't know how to handle things.

My home life and support network was an ocean away – fifteen hours by plane. Trying to make the right decisions for all my employees and my family's future, I was worrying about my babies and missing home at the same time. In Australia I was considered super responsible, but in LA I felt like a kid chasing rainbows, looking for some pot of gold.

I knew I needed to make connections, but who to trust? Everyone there positions themselves as super important and it's easy to be fooled by what they say. I got swindled by some people who made huge promises around Tammy Fit. Already connected with them as a supplier, I trusted them to help us with the app and paid them in advance. But they never delivered and I lost *a lot* of money.

It's easy to look back at that experience and berate myself. But I was young and naive enough to still believe that people have your best interests at heart. Now I'm more careful. There's horrible greed in the world – it exists anywhere a lot of money is involved – and I'm a lot more wary of it now. I like to think that the older, wiser version of me would have known to take precautions and triple-check everything, but perhaps she would have been taken advantage of too. I think it was made worse at the time by my head and heart being in overwhelm. Regardless, it was a big lesson in trust.

I lost my innocence from that experience. I've learnt that people will lie to your face, will tell you exactly what you want to hear and that you can't take them on face value. You *must* do your own due diligence. No matter what you think you know, or how much you value the person you're dealing with, you *must* bring in expert advice, legal advice too. Otherwise, you leave yourself, your staff and your family vulnerable.

We're all born with an open heart and as babies we have no choice but to trust in others to care for us. You could say that having trust is our natural state. It makes it easy at first, but once you've been betrayed like that? It's much harder. Sadly, not all lessons in life make you happier, some of them just make you smarter and more wary. And maybe as we evolve, the independence and self-belief we develop from surviving those ordeals is a good thing. We *are* happy, it's just a new kind of happy. I'll never be that innocent, naive, over-trusting young girl again. But I am a strong woman who takes care of herself and her own, and no-one can take that away from me. Now that my heart is stronger, there's more of it to give.

Having your trust broken hurts. A lot. In the aftermath, it's important to nurture yourself back to a safe state. It's easy to blame yourself, but what's the use in that? It's vital to take ownership, sure. If we don't learn from our mistakes, we're destined to repeat them. But carrying shame for a mistake made simply because we didn't know better? That doesn't help anyone. Shame says 'I am bad' whereas guilt separates the person from the behaviour: 'I did something bad.' Take the lesson, apologise and make amends if you need to, then move forward with your head held high and heart open.

Let it go

In the long run, those who persistently lie, cheat and deceive will be left carrying the burden of shame. There is no guilt in making an honest mistake. If you're still carrying some hurt over broken trust, here's a reflection for you:

This is why I am glad I was the one who trusted and not the other way around:

....

....

....

It says this about my heart:

....

....

....

It has taught me this:

....

....

....

I can look in the mirror and tell myself that I am (these loving words):

....

....

....

The easiest way
to get lost is to
forget what you
were looking for.

DAZZLING
LA LIGHTS

Sooner or later, life gets . . . tempting. As it should. At some point, we must push beyond our comfort zone to learn where our personal boundaries lie. How else do we determine our limits? When that's on a Hollywood scale, the temptations are supernova – experiences of a lifetime. It's an aspirational lifestyle, so when you're extended a hand, you don't say no. No promises you won't get burnt, though.

If you're pushed beyond your safe space it can be difficult to locate your intuition. The external world gets *very* loud and the future looks *very* bright. Blinding, in fact. It's easy to lose your way.

*

With my life split between LA and Australia, my world was spinning on several axes. I was mothering toddlers, reeling from a relationship break-up, negotiating with finance sharks, growing two businesses, travelling across oceans. I don't think I've ever been that exhausted and stretched in my life. I needed something positive to reach for. Friends who could understand this exhilarating new landscape I was navigating.

233

Some high-profile celebrities reached out to me and soon I was modelling for them. By the time I was on my third campaign, we had become friends. My life had been exciting before, but this world was next level. I was regularly mixing with the rich and famous and was brought into their incredible lifestyles. There were endless parties and fashion shows, glitz and glamour all heaving with celebrities. Travelling by private jet became standard.

Although I was used to my life being scrutinised, mingling in this scene took it up several notches. The media loved that I had become part of the LA scene and the press loves a good angle, so they pushed it hard. Since most people in Hollywood keep their real lives incredibly private, the photojournalists will do anything to generate a story. Even if it's patently untrue. The industry and world surrounding it is filled with smoke and mirrors, the line between truth and fiction easily blurred.

Hello, is it me you're looking for?

Have you ever found yourself so deep into a new project, job or social group, you've lost sight of your original goal and true self? It's easy to get caught up in the noise of a new world and forget your inner truths. Try to remember when this has happened to you and spend some time writing about it. Journalling, unfiltered, can unearth unexpected insights.

....

....

....

....

I've had negative things said about me and there have been times when I've cried to my sister, can I please just go defend myself? But she talks me down and says, no, it's not worth it. And I'm glad. I'm so glad we've always been like that.

Sometimes,
something has
to give.

THAT PARTY

'Make hay while the sun shines' we're told. Living in Australia, we know only too well how the weather can affect a harvest. Beyond farming, this motto rings true for anyone looking to grow their business. Mine is no different. When I had successfully launched Tammy Fit and Saski and was being pulled into the LA orbit, all my education, training and instinct told me to *lean in*. I was surrounded by great examples of how to successfully turn a personal brand into a thriving enterprise.

*

As part of the LA glitz and glam, I was invited to an exclusive party. A huge part of me was excited. But I had just got home from a work trip and, although I often took them with me, for this one, my kids had stayed home. All I really wanted to do was snuggle with them and have some playtime. But work was as busy as ever and really needed my attention. I was torn.

I talked it through with my sisters and made the call. This event was something I didn't want to miss and I knew it would be a quick trip that my heart and work would both benefit from.

I packed my bags and flew to LA. By the time I landed, I hadn't slept for thirty hours. Exiting the plane, I felt horribly jet-lagged and like a zombie, but there was no time to rest. I went straight into hair and make-up and getting dressed. I was completely exhausted and kept falling asleep in the make-up chair. My heart was aching from my recent break-up and I was missing my kids more than ever, but this was important. I pulled myself together and headed to the party.

I was still a relative newcomer to the LA scene. Getting to know people takes effort and my friends had yet to arrive, so I walked through the crowd and chatted. I took a drink or two as they were offered, no more than usual. One minute I was fine, but in the next, I was not okay. Then all of a sudden, I collapsed.

I don't remember the paparazzi. I don't remember being taken out in front of all of those cameras. My whole world came crashing down.

If at first you don't listen . . .

I only have a very simple activity at this point: read and reflect upon this quote. I read it not long after this terrible moment. It makes so much sense to me. It is so, so true.

'Make time for rest or your body will force you to slow down in ways you probably won't like.'

So basically what happened was that I was in LA running on pretty much 30 hours of no sleep. I was struggling to stay awake, even when I was getting my hair & make-up done and I could barely keep my eyes open. I think because of the break-up I've been trying to keep myself busy and not really taking time to think about how I'm actually feeling or focusing on myself.

I probably shouldn't have been drinking considering how jet-lagged and how exhausted I was and I already wasn't feeling well . . . so yeah, I pretty much collapsed. I'm already super, super embarrassed about it.

I've been throwing myself into work way more than ever and I have my kids the majority of the time . . . literally been non-stop on the job kind of thing . . . it's not my finest moment . . .

When you hit
rock bottom, the
only way is up.

A VERY
PUBLIC CRISIS

I don't know if you've ever hit rock bottom. By this point, I thought I knew what a crisis felt like. I'd survived my parents' divorce, banished those dark times pre-Tammy Fit and had been suffering post-break-up. But crises take many forms. There's the slow burning type of crisis, when things aren't going well for a long time, such as my uni years; then there's the heartache of break-up, which is excruciating and personal but somewhat private. And then there's this: a very sudden, very public crisis . . . I was *not* prepared.

*

Opening your eyes and finding yourself in hospital is bad. Realising you have a headache, no, *raging* hangover, is bad. Not remembering how you got there is bad. But when I checked my phone and began scrolling . . . bad became *terrifying*. The coverage was insane. Every new post felt like a king hit.

The pictures were plastered *everywhere*. Followed by vitriolic hatred from online trolls. A tidal wave of abuse, literally thousands and thousands of messages filled with condemnation.

I was accused of taking drugs – I didn't. Of drinking copious amounts of alcohol – I didn't. Of being a social climber. Of

... people trolling or being nasty or making up things just for no good reason. I mean, I personally could never imagine attacking someone or judging someone for something like this. You just never know what someone is going through. It's a reminder to be kind always. There are people who go through worse things than this, at the end of the day.

abusing my privilege. That I was disgusting, the lowest person alive. That I had no morals, no values.

Perhaps I could have handled it better if I wasn't already in a vulnerable place. Perhaps, if I had deserved it.

But I was twenty-four, far from home and the people who loved me. I had no safety barrier between me and the haters – tens upon tens of thousands of them – and they wouldn't let up. Suddenly, I felt very young. Very alone. And a failure.

This was my rock bottom. My breaking point. I curled up in a ball and cried and cried and cried. I didn't think I would ever stop. I'd been so strong for so long, pushed through so many obstacles. I'd fought my way through depression, the naysayers, the deniers, financial abuse, heartbreak. But I was broken. Spent.

I wanted to speak out, but doubted anyone would believe me. I felt loathed, ostracised and discarded. The reality of my recent break-up hit me with new force. I was utterly alone.

In that moment, it felt like the whole world hated me. In an instant, I'd gone from media darling to public enemy number one. The press and public wouldn't stop tearing me down; they were like bloodthirsty animals. The thick skin I had built up over the years became cellophane.

After some painful soul searching, questioning whether they were right, whether I deserved to be alone, I looked up. I hadn't got to this point in my life by being a victim. If I had believed the things people said about me, I would never have had Wolf, never started my businesses or had my beautiful daughters. I wouldn't have the incredible success and happiness I had built for myself and my family.

Family. My bedrock. The people I knew who loved me, no matter what. Despite the many mistakes I have made, the questionable decisions I have taken, the annoying traits I undoubtedly have, they *always* have my back.

I picked up the phone. They were there. 'Come home, sis,' they said. 'We've got you.'

I'd lost my way in LA looking for what I already had. The worst thing had happened, but it opened my eyes to the truth. I packed my bags and flew in the direction of love.

When the worst hits

When you hit rock bottom, remember this:

1. If this is the worst, it has to get better from here. The only way is up.

2. Reach out to those who love you, they will carry you when you can't carry yourself.

3. Being hard on yourself won't fix things. Being kind to yourself and self-healing will.

4. One day, you may learn from this. Focus on getting well and trust that something better may come.

Stop chasing
stuff and just
appreciate
what's real.

WHERE THE
HEART IS

They say it's not what *happens* to you, but how you *deal* with it. Also, what you *learn* from it. If you don't pick up the lesson, life has a funny habit of delivering it to you over and again, until you do.

*

LA now feels like a fever dream, one that ended in a nightmare. Yet I don't feel sorry for that twenty-four-year-old me. Looking back, I learnt so much from that period. As hard as it was, it was such an incredible growth opportunity. Self-pity is so pointless. It just makes you feel worse. It's easy to get sucked into others' warped opinions of you, but they're not real.

With perspective, I look at younger me with tenderness. She was a kid with big dreams and thought she'd find them on the City of Angels' glittering boulevards. I won't be the first or last to tell that story. Amazing things happen in LA, but some really dark stuff happens too. While short trips are great for my businesses, I prefer to live my life here in Australia. This is home.

All this perspective and learning didn't happen overnight. I had a moment of clarity the next day, but I had a long way to go from there. The mean haze of the fallout stuck around for a while. But slowly, the love of my children, my sisters, friends and family helped me heal. I used to care so much more about what people said and thought about me. The horror of the LA party aftermath showed me that what the trolls and the media think of you doesn't actually matter. They are strangers. They don't know you. The opinion of a person who loves you far outweighs them all.

There's another old saying that I like: what doesn't kill you makes you stronger. I have my mental and physical health. I have love. That's worth showing up for – the only thing worth showing up for, when it comes down to it. I don't do what I do for the money or the accolades. I do it for my children, my family, my friends, my community. I do it for love.

Chasing pots of gold at the ends of distant rainbows is an illusion. Why chase stuff when you can appreciate what's right in front of you – what's *real*? So I do that now, on my terms, with people I trust. I still have ambition and I'm always building on what I have. But these days it's in a happy way, with balance.

That was a big lesson. You can achieve extraordinary things, but you'll be far happier focusing on the few things that really matter and getting those right. Being content with your version of 'having it all' is far better than trying to have too much.

Self-pity is one of the most destructive attitudes you can have. I honestly think it's one of the worst things you can do – to throw yourself a pity party and feel sorry for yourself . . . play the victim, that kind of thing. I believe that you should focus on self-compassion and gratitude instead. In most situations, there's still always things that you could be grateful for, like simply waking up in the morning. That is a huge thing to be grateful for! Breathe the air into your lungs and be grateful for just that! Practising gratitude is key and it's something you have to do again and again. You need to consistently consider how lucky are to wake up each day. Life is the greatest privilege there is.

Big lessons

What big life lessons have you learnt? I think they're more important than any kind of formal learning. 'Degrees of the heart' I call
them – they require way more effort than any uni degree and deliver
far richer results. List a few of yours here:

....

....

....

....

It's better to be
kind than to
be right.

LET IT BE

Regardless of all the life lessons we're willing to learn, sometimes things remain stuck. What do you do when, despite all your effort, you can't change them?

When you really think about it, 'stuckness' is often just a matter of opinion. As an influencer I cop a lot of unsolicited 'advice' about my personal life. People say, 'Sticks and stones will break your bones but words will never hurt you.' They also say, 'Words are mightier than the sword.' Which one is true? Both. The secret is knowing whose words to listen to and whose to ignore.

*

These days, I'm much better at ignoring the haters, but when I was starting out, I used to get hurt really easily. Since it's basically part of my job, I had to learn, pretty quickly, how not to let them get to me.

If I notice I'm feeling hurt or sad about something that's been said, the first thing I do is take a step back. I observe my emotions rather than let them take over. It can be hard in the heat of the moment, so tricks like trying to describe them in words, how they feel and where they're located in my body, can be helpful.

It helps me calm down and gives me space to reflect. Most of all, it helps me avoid those knee-jerk reactions of the past. Instead of getting overwhelmed by the emotion, I sit with it. After the intensity subsides, I can reframe the situation in my mind.

Who honestly cares what those trolls think? If they could do what I do, they would, or if not, at least pursue their own equivalent passion. Instead they hide behind their words, trying to make someone else feel bad because they hate their own life. Anyone who has time to spend bitching about others clearly doesn't have much going on. I feel sorry for them.

It reminds me to forget about them and focus on my own life. When I set my intention and pour my energies into my own goals, I don't have time to worry about what other people say. When I'm making progress, I couldn't care less what they think. My actions speak far louder than their words. Every forward step I take gets me further and further away from their petty hates and petty opinions.

If the message is too ugly to ignore, or could send the wrong message to my community, then I don't retreat to my corner. Once again, I take action. I might post a reply to clarify things or release a public statement if it needs a serious response. Mostly, I prefer not to give them air time. These bullies are just looking for attention, so generally, I'd rather not give it to them. Firing back only prolongs the argument and trying to prove you're right is guaranteed to fail. They're not willing to listen, no matter how much you try to explain yourself.

I feel angry when I read those messages, sure, but I prefer the saying, 'It's better to be kind than right.' I don't mean you should reach out and be all sweetness and light – we've already established trolls are only in it for themselves. But you could be kind by trying to understand that perhaps their circumstances have created a bitterness in them, and you can feel some empathy. But don't engage. Instead, be kind to yourself. Just let it go. People will have their perspective; be at peace with that.

Step back and reflect

If others' words and opinions get to you, follow these steps to create some space.

1. Stand back, pause and observe.

2. Reflect on what's happening, don't react.

3. Believe in yourself.

4. Don't get drawn into the drama.

5. It's better to be kind than right.

6. Let. It. Be.

... continue to live with only love and softness in your heart, no matter what cards you are dealt and how hard the world tries to make you.

DEVELOPMENT

Life changes constantly. Fight it all you like, but everything is temporary. If you don't keep rolling with the tides, you'll either get swamped or left ashore. But there's no value in swimming through life like a zombie-fish with your eyes and ears clammed shut. If you go with the flow but fail to learn the lesson, it will come back to bite you again, and again, until you do. In other words, whether you like it or not, we're all here to learn and grow.

There's no point hiding from hard things. They'll push you out of your comfort zone, which may hurt a little, but pushing is *good*. Beyond the boundaries is where growth is found. After every major obstacle you overcome, the person you were before has changed. You learnt. You grew. You had to. Good.

You won't be doing this alone. For some of us, our greatest challenge is learning how to accept help. Equally important is recognising others. Making people feel valued and important. Seen. No-one likes to be overlooked! Paying complete attention to the moment you're in and the person you're with is key. Living in the now. It's powerful.

To get the most from each moment, you must know what drives you. What's important to you and what makes you happy.

Every phase in life is temporary.
Embrace every moment. When
life is good, be sure to enjoy it &
receive it fully. When life is tough,
remember that it too will pass.

When, how, why, where and to whom you give your time should be guided by this. Otherwise you're letting others dictate how you spend your life. You only get one. Make it count.

Finding a balance across all areas is fundamental. This book addresses eight key sectors and, in this section, I'll share how I spread my energy and help you design where to focus yours. Balance is critical, but you'll only find this once you've worked out what you value most and want to pay attention to. What works for me, or my sisters, won't necessarily work for you. It's also likely to change as you move through life and your priorities shift.

From everything I've experienced and learnt along the way, I'm happy to share some of my secrets to ongoing growth and development. Many of these I learnt through the books in my step-dad's library, others from wise friends, but I learnt the most from my personal experiences – good and bad. I've learnt one thing above all: how to make choices that are good for the *soul*.

There's no
point in hiding
from the hard
things - they'll
always find you.

HIDE AND SEEK

We so often like to hide from hard things, because why would we choose to run headlong into pain? Well, when it comes to being the best version of yourself, there's no better fast track. The longer I've lived, the more I've learnt to *willingly* walk towards challenges. Now, I embrace them because I know how much stronger I'll be on the other side. It wasn't always that way.

I used to avoid speechmaking like the plague. Hated it. As I mentioned earlier, despite being a public figure, I'm actually quite shy. Doing interviews or public-speaking events has always felt seriously painful. Yet, I make myself do them anyway. Why? Because it's part of my job. You can't sign up to stuff then only do the things that please you. Every gig has its challenges and being an influencer is no different. If you're not prepared to put in the hard work and do the difficult things, then don't expect to get anywhere.

It can be excruciating and your body will send out crazy signals – *don't do it!* Unless you're in genuine danger, ignore them. It just our mind's way of telling our body it doesn't like this. When it comes to pushing ourselves out of our comfort zone, our minds turn us into wobbling jelly legs. *Not* helpful. Much like observing your emotions, observing these physical sensations and reminding yourself that they are simply symptoms of a healthy nervous system can help keep us focused. It can help, again, to describe the physical sensations you're feeling and locate them in your body. Thank your mind for alerting you to danger, then tell it to stand down. *You've got this.*

*

As a parent, one of the proudest moments is when you know your kid is scared of doing something, but does it anyway. When they start at a new school, sing in front of assembly, or stand up to a bully. Though wary, most kids tend to jump straight in, but as we get older, we start to overthink things.

We worry about all the things that might go wrong, who we might hurt in the process, where we could end up. The longer we think, the more scenarios we create. But guess what – only *one* of them can come true! It doesn't matter how many alternatives you lay out for yourself, in the end, *only one will happen.* The rest will live in your imagination forever, begun wild and gone to seed. Meanwhile, your tea's gone cold and someone else has already launched that product.

I've found that the more you dwell on something, the harder you make it for yourself. Even going to do a workout, if I sit and procrastinate over whether I should go, start imagining all the hard things about it, I can put myself off completely and won't go. By the time I've run through the workout in my head and imagined all the effort, I could have been halfway through! What a waste. So I don't give myself that opportunity. I just get up and go without even thinking about it.

It's easy to talk yourself out of doing that hard thing by imagining scary possibilities, but reality will nearly always work out far better than you think. By sitting there daydreaming, you're depriving yourself of an opportunity to chase something wonderful. All that energy spent tossing ideas around could have been put into creating something. Anything.

Taking action is guaranteed to deliver results. You may not always like them, but at least you'll have something to work with. Then you take the next step and the next. Soon enough you'll have landed where you wanted – maybe even *further* ahead. So stop daydreaming and start doing! You never know what's around the corner until you physically show up.

Get real with yourself

Are you avoiding something 'hard' even though you know you would benefit from doing it? Maybe it's a course or applying for a job promotion or starting a new exercise routine or going on a date. Ask yourself these questions:

What are you avoiding?

But what are you *really* hiding from?

What's the worst thing that could happen? How likely is that?

What's the best thing that could happen? Is that probable?

What is the most likely thing to happen if you did this?

What achievable step can you take towards it?

*Ask yourself:
is that really
true?*

I BELIEVE . . . ?

What's stopping you from seeking in the first place? Many behaviours are directed by underlying beliefs we've held for so long, we don't even see them anymore. The identity they have created is 'just who we are'. At least, that's the story we tell ourselves.

Many of our internal beliefs are formed in childhood as a way of navigating the world. They're often fear-based, which is natural, if they developed as a protective measure. You soon learn to make yourself quiet if you're yelled at often enough, small if you are not given space, or wilfully blind if questioning authority is punished.

But since then, you have grown. Your world has changed. You're an adult with far more agency than in childhood. You can create your own life, based on your own dreams. But first, you must believe that they are possible.

Those who held us back in childhood are no longer in charge, yet we carry their directives into our future. We came to believe the stories we were told and continue to operate under their direction. We've developed so much negative self-talk that it holds us back, but if we look to the origin of those beliefs, it's just fear. The things that we worry 'might' happen, are only a bunch of possibilities. Most of them won't materialise, yet we let fear win, every time. We let the ghosts under the bed come out to play. And so, the story continues.

*

As a young girl, I was frequently described as 'shy'. Sure, I was quieter than some. I didn't much like being called on to answer a question, or speaking in front of the class, or giving my opinion to a bunch of adults. People would excuse me as being 'shy' and so I started to believe it. *I'm quiet. I'm shy. I hate being put on the spot. I hate speaking in front of people. I'm no good at it.*

Yet as it turns out, despite my so-called shyness, I've actually become pretty good at speaking up! I've been invited to appear at big events all around the world. I regularly announce to camera. I am the spokesperson for my brands. And you'd better believe I'll stand up for my kids whenever they need it. I'm not shy, I just don't need to be the centre of attention. Unless it means something. Unless I need to.

Underlying beliefs develop from moments of self-doubt, from a thoughtless passing comment, even from people thinking they're being kind. It doesn't matter their intention, it just matters what you hear, believe and internalise. Once those beliefs take root, they can make you want to hide away, afraid to show what you can do. Old beliefs are often no more than a line you feed yourself. *I am lazy, I am too loud, I'm embarrassing, I can't stand up for myself, I never have anything interesting to say, I'm terrible at relationships, I'm gullible, I'm poor, I always say the wrong thing.* It's frightening how much we can believe them to be true. But they're just stories. Just lines. Often lies.

You may have inherited some beliefs from your family or the wider culture. Beliefs around achievements, roles and responsibilities: 'a house by twenty-seven', 'retire at sixty', 'you can't have a baby at nineteen', or 'women can't run businesses'. Who says? Because it's 'always been that way'? Well not anymore, buddy. Not on my watch.

'Comparisonitis' is huge these days, especially being able to compare ourselves across social media. If you're inspired to go after more, great. But not at the expense of your health. Not if it doesn't align with your values. Not if it's not what will make *you* happy.

You can't worry about what others think. I've seen so many people hold themselves back because they're too worried about someone else's opinion. These underlying beliefs are sneaky too, because often they masquerade as your own thoughts. If you really stopped to examine them and asked where they've come from and whether they truly hold water, you'd realise a lot of them are inherited.

The real danger is when they stop you going after what you want. If they are driven by fear, then you're letting fear hold you back: *I can't!*

I'm here to tell you that you *can*. You can if you believe you can. So examine your beliefs and decide if they are still true for you. See which ones you might want to change, then set about changing them. What you believe will come true, so make sure you believe in the right things.

Examine your internal beliefs

Are you carrying around old beliefs that are holding you back? Fill in this chart to find out.

A limiting thought	Where it came from	How I could move forward
I never finish things.	Dropping out of school.	Enrolling in something new.

Never be the
smartest person
in the room.

THE GIFT OF BEING PRESENT

Everyone has a message for you. Everyone has a story, offers something you can learn. A favourite Hembrow saying is, 'If you're the smartest person in the room, you're in the wrong room.' You don't want to stay dormant in life, you want to progress and grow. Don't sit at home by yourself, disconnected. Get out there, meet people, try new things, open your mind and keep growing.

You can let life's moments and people pass you by, but it's far more interesting to make each count. How? Focus! Being present for the person in front of you is one of the most-practised habits of highly successful people. For a start, it's polite. Second, it's a gift that runs both ways. When you are one-on-one with someone it's an opportunity for a private, personal exchange. Yet so many of us waste that. We're scrolling on our phones, or watching TV, or keeping an eye out for the tennis score.

Taking time to prioritise each person in front of you and giving them your full attention is key. It makes you an *active* listener, so you'll absorb far more of what they're saying – and you never know what pearls of wisdom you might take home. You're also valuing them, showing them they *matter*. This will deepen your connection. And who knows where that might take you?

Something so special about the connection we all have. We all share this human experience. We all share in feeling human emotions. Love, joy, sadness, loss. We all go through things, good and bad. We're all connected in that way. And I hope that if you're ever feeling lonely, you remember that. We're not as different as you think. 🫶

*

Think about the most impressive people you've met and I can almost guarantee they're the ones who fully focus on you when you talk. You find yourself saying things you didn't expect to share. That's because these people are *invested* in you. Their focus says 'you matter to me more than anyone else in this room right at this moment', and that's about the greatest compliment you can pay someone. It's also smart.

Dale Carnegie's *How to Win Friends and Influence People* says to talk in terms of other people's interests because that's usually what they're most passionate about. I already know all about my own life, so I don't need to hear about that again. I learn so much more listening to other people: what they've experienced, how they've built businesses, navigated romance, even which new movies they've loved!

Meeting preparation

I value meeting people so much that I prepare myself before I go out. When building connections, here are my two tips:

1. **Take a minute beforehand.** It's really worthwhile to pause before you enter an event or meeting to *shake off everything weighing on your mind* and leave it at the door. Taking a few deep and calming breaths helps you to walk in fresh and revived with your full focus on what's ahead.

2. **Bring a clear head.** When it comes to being alert, being active helps. My schedule is extremely busy and changes daily, but if I can't keep to my morning gym routine, I always try to set an hour aside each day to exercise in some way. With a clear head, I find it so much easier to feel present in my body and connected to those around me.

List the ways in which you mentally prepare to meet with people.

....

....

....

....

....

....

Design the life you enjoy.

A WELL-DESIGNED LIFE

Yes, you can design the life you want, but there are no guarantees it will go to plan. Yet having your goals and action steps set out is valuable because it helps keep you focused. I love my weekly routine. It's been handpicked for me, by me. If you're already wishing your day was over before it begins, it might pay to review your schedule. Even if, right now, you're committed to a job that pays the bills, by reviewing your schedule, you could create time to develop new skills for a better future, or more fun with friends to counteract all those long, boring days. That's where having a routine is invaluable – it will stop you wasting time and help you spend it on the important things.

These days, I've designed my life so that I'm excited about each and every thing on my to-do list. Enjoying your routine is important, because if you like it, you'll do it. Even the harder things, like an early morning ab workout, are welcome because I have chosen them. I know they're positive uses of my time. I know I'm working towards my personal goals, my ongoing big dream, and that feels motivating and amazing. Plus you get an endorphin buzz after working out and feel energised and strong. My routine ensures I have plenty of time for the kids, work and socialising. There's room for spontaneity (always) and fun (always, always) and of course, the Hembrow village.

*

My current weekly ritual looks pretty much like this. Remember, this is what works for *me* and it's only an example. Hopefully it will spark ideas for you.

	Monday to Friday	Saturday to Sunday
Early	*5 a.m.* Wake up, do my skincare routine and read while I have a coffee. *5.30 a.m.* 20 to 30 minutes of yoga, Pilates, or meditation. *6 a.m.* My kids wake up and we start the hustle and bustle of the school morning.	Sleep in when I can – Posy is still quite young and gets up early!
Morning	*7 a.m.* Make kids' breakfast, lunches and pack for school. *9 a.m.* Meet with my team and PA and start the day.	*7 a.m.* Get up with kids, breakfast and playtime. *9 a.m.* Pack for the day's adventures.

	Monday to Friday	**Saturday to Sunday**
Day	*9 a.m.–5 p.m.* Run Tammy Fit and Saski, including meetings, photoshoots, designing, strategising, emailing, networking, as well as running around after one very cheeky baby.	*No set times* – just a day of adventuring at the beach or movies or picnicking or sport.
Afternoon	*5 p.m.–6 p.m.* Homework, reading, music practice and a little TV while I cook everyone dinner.	
Evening	*6 p.m.–8 p.m.* Bath time then a movie or reading books in Mummy's room.	*Saturday* Unless I have an event or a party it's family and close friends celebration time at my place!
After dinner	*8 p.m.–10 p.m.* Tucking in, then once they're all in bed for the night, I catch up on any laundry/last-minute work, then usually I have some Netflix or book time for myself.	*Sunday* Family dinner then wind down. Get uniforms ready and organised for the week ahead.

Review your time
Now it's your turn! Fill in the blank weekly chart below to see how
you are currently spending your time, then consider where you could
tweak things to design the life you want.

	Monday to Friday	Saturday to Sunday
Early		
Morning		
Day		
Afternoon		
Evening		
After dinner		

Notes:

....

....

....

Like feeding a plant, mind-food will help you grow.

SELF-DEVELOPMENT, IT'S PERSONAL

We have so much to learn about ourselves and so much potential. No-one on this earth is perfect – there is *always* room for growth. I don't want to be some sad neglected pot plant in the corner wilting away. I want to be strong and flourish through all seasons, grow tall and proud, like a rainforest palm. To reach our full potential, we need nourishment and challenges. In forest management, hazard-reduction burns encourage new growth – the healthy response to trauma. The more work you put in, the more you'll get out. So make like nature and be a tree.

*

There are several ways I prioritise self-development. Books are my foundation. I love to read and a motivational book will always inspire me. I highlight sentences and mark pages as I go. Re-reading a good book is like visiting an old friend, it reinforces key messages, plus you'll always glean something new based on what's important to you at the time.

Podcasts, audiobooks and online articles are also a great source of info. As are people. I'm a big fan of asking questions. Ask, ask, ask! There are *no* stupid questions and answers come from the strangest places. When I first started out, Google

Meditating really changed my life. One of the first times I tried it, I got into a deep meditation & had a full out-of-body experience, completely disconnected from my physical being, and there was really no looking back from there. I decided then, I would dedicate my life to becoming the healthiest, happiest version of myself. Meditating for even just 10 minutes a day can help relieve stress, calm your mind & clear it of negative thoughts, and help you really focus on the present. ⸎ There's no doubt in my mind, meditation has helped me, not just in daily life but even in my businesses & creativity.

was helpful. A real-life mentor is unbeatable. Networking, events and conferences provide opportunities to meet people and connect. Surrounding yourself with like-minded folk generates an amazing energy. No matter where I go, I always meet new, interesting people. I make it my priority to *connect*.

I believe in breaking goals down into achievable steps, but often our goals hold future dreams. If you've never done something, how do you know what steps to take? Ask people who have. People love to share their success and good fortune. Ask them what worked and what didn't, what they might do differently, what their key piece of advice is for someone starting out. We are all a work in progress and there's nothing like inspiration to fuel you.

My final word on personal development is to *make it personal*. We're each motivated by different things, so find what works for you and use it. I use post-it notes, Emilee uses her phone screen, Amy uses LinkedIn. If you read a motivational quote, message it to yourself. If you see something that inspires you, take a photo. If a song speaks to your heart, add it to your playlist. The more positive inputs you add to your brain, the more those messages will sink in. Mind-food. Like feeding a plant, it will help you grow.

Your personal inspiration

Make your own self-development power list of personal inspirations:

- Books

- Journals

- Podcasts

- Music

If it's good for the soul, do it more.

JOYFUL MOMENTS

Everything I do involves passion, but not everything can be my top priority. Some things I love doing, but they can't be my number one focus. Every so often I try to make time for them because they light up my soul. Life is huge and filled with possibility. New ideas are often sparked by new experiences. So get out and try something different. Have fun and who knows what you'll dream up along the way.

*

For a start, I love fashion. I've been obsessed with clothes and shoe shopping ever since I was little. Cruising around online retail for ten minutes is therapy for me. I also love getting a facial or a massage – luckily, my sisters run a skin clinic! There's nothing quite like girl time.

Music is a huge part of my life. I'm always singing, even when I speak. My playlist is long and I'm always updating it. I love movies too – movie nights with my family are the best. We're always having fun, being silly and doing arts and craft around at home. I love travelling with them too. Being out in nature is soul food for me. Sunshine or rain, the beach, mountains or rainforest, sunrise or sunset. I feel at peace outside.

It's so important to spend time unplugged. Off the screens, big and small. My work can be non-stop – running my own companies means I don't have set hours, so it's easy to get stuck on the phone or laptop. It can feel easier to give the kids their own screens to keep them occupied. So I'm mindful of limiting that – for them *and* me. I don't want my kids to spend huge chunks of their childhoods in artificial worlds. And I don't want to miss out on these precious years of family time because I'm always working. As a rule, we have time outdoors every day with plenty of active and imaginative playtime.

My other big family rule is a strict one: no working for me on weekends. On Saturdays and Sundays, I focus solely on my children and don't allow any distractions from work to interfere. Instead, I pack the car and we head out for a day of adventure. It can be hard, especially if something is urgent. But I remind myself that it isn't going anywhere and can be done on Monday. What's most important is enjoying life and spending time with my kids in the real world.

Part-time passions

What are your side passions – the little things that make your heart sing? Write a list and see if you can add a few more joyful moments to your days.

....

....

....

Happiest place. 🌊 Salt water is so healing. Sweat, tears & the sea. 👻👻

Balance is all about weighing up what works for you.

BALANCING
THE PIE

The ultimate goal of self-development is to create a life you *love*. A big part of that is getting the *balance* right. Time management plays a huge role here. Not only what you add to your schedule, but also what you eliminate. I've spent a lot of time thinking about the things I don't want in my life and actively removing them from my week so I can fill it with more of the things I do.

Getting the balance right across all areas of life is key. Focus too much on one area at the expense of another, and pretty soon you'll start to feel it. You may notice you're more grumpy or down than usual, that your spark is missing, that you feel lonely. Your mind is telling you your balance is off. Perhaps you've been partying so hard, your health is faltering. Giving all your attention to your career and not enough time to friends. If you've stopped calling them back or checking in with them, chances are they'll do the same. An easy fix? Make time for them. Redress the balance.

*

I'm continuously reviewing my schedule and routines to ensure that the kids and I are getting the balance right. I'm far from perfect and often things have to change if I'm travelling or launching a new product. The same goes if it's the beginning or end of the school year when it seems like there's some sort of event every other day. Mapping out my ideal life helps remind me of what's important and brings me back on track if things swerve. That's life. So long as I'm keeping the balance right most of the time, then that in itself is balance. Your ideal balance will be completely different from mine, so just use it as a guide to develop your own.

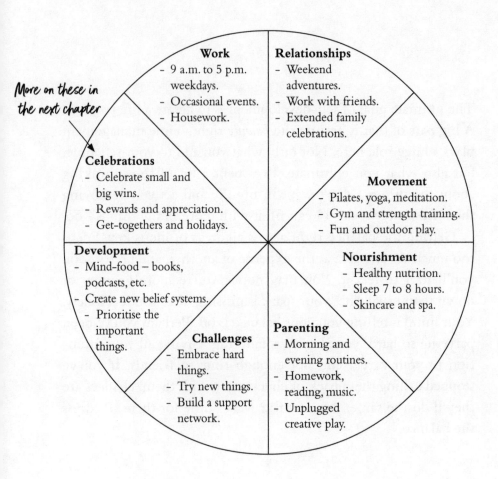

More on these in the next chapter

Work
- 9 a.m. to 5 p.m. weekdays.
- Occasional events.
- Housework.

Relationships
- Weekend adventures.
- Work with friends.
- Extended family celebrations.

Celebrations
- Celebrate small and big wins.
- Rewards and appreciation.
- Get-togethers and holidays.

Movement
- Pilates, yoga, meditation.
- Gym and strength training.
- Fun and outdoor play.

Development
- Mind-food – books, podcasts, etc.
- Create new belief systems.
- Prioritise the important things.

Nourishment
- Healthy nutrition.
- Sleep 7 to 8 hours.
- Skincare and spa.

Challenges
- Embrace hard things.
- Try new things.
- Build a support network.

Parenting
- Morning and evening routines.
- Homework, reading, music.
- Unplugged creative play.

Your ideal life

Your turn! Add an equal amount of activities to each category to support your well-balanced life.

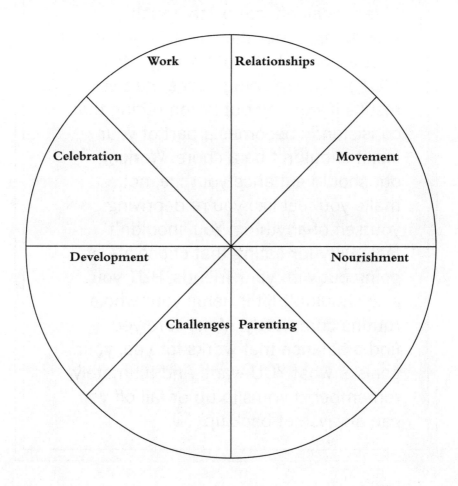

Let's talk about BALANCE. ⚖️ My approach to fitness is never about being 'all consumed' by it. (For example, I literally had the WHOLE of last week off, ate pretty much everything under the sun, lots of fine cheeses, sweets & spicy margaritas 🌶️🍸). You are going to see the best results if working out is something that consistently becomes a part of your life, it shouldn't be a chore. Working out should enhance your life, not make you feel like you're depriving yourself of anything. You shouldn't feel guilty for eating that chocolate or going out with your friends, BUT you also shouldn't let it derail your whole routine completely. Make sure you find a balance that works for you, your goals & what YOU want. And ultimately, remember, if you slip up or fall off you can always get back up. 😊

CELEBRATION

From all that overwhelm I learnt that life needs to be celebrated *now*. Use the picnic hamper, crack open the champagne, serve those nibbles on the good china and burn the scented candles. It's all there to be used, not hidden away – and so is all that joy inside you!

Celebration takes many forms. It's parties and streamers, but it's also everyday occasions. Unboxing a new purchase, savouring a smoothie, enjoying a mid-week pedicure, giving a back tickle. Celebrate small wins, like completing your workout; and big wins like getting a pay rise! 'We time' or 'me time', they're *all* good.

Celebrations happen within. The best thing about internal parties? They can happen anywhere, anytime. Between you and your giddy heart, let's get this party started. Turn on joy. Appreciate what's right in front of you – life is good *right now*! Reflect on a past win – there's always something joyful to remember. There's no limit to internal celebrations. No-one's watching, no-one's counting, so go crazy!

Celebrations are rewards – for you and anyone else who deserves recognition. Gifts, bonuses, commendations, prizes, accolades, decorations, medals. Personally, I like them in the way of dollars, chocolates, flowers and trips. Awards are nice too. At home and at work. Giving can feel better than receiving.

Celebrations are holidays. The festive holidays at home with all the trimmings, the family holidays we take, the work trips I have, the people I meet. I love travelling; opening my eyes, my heart and soul to new people and places. That's what I call a celebration.

Celebration can be living it up, living it humble, living it loud, living it soft. Celebration is the stuff of life – embracing the best of everything. Without celebration, what is the point? Don't wait for weddings or birthdays or Christmas. Do it more. Do it *daily*.

Today was just so surreal. 🫧🐬 Watching baby dolphins flipping in the air. Snorkelling with sharks. Blessed to be able to share these experiences with my little humans. 🥹 Our cups r fulllll.

Big things take
up a lot of room,
but it's the little
things that
count.

THE SMALL WINS

Progress is often measured in milestones – first steps, completing a subject, saving a house deposit. But the little steps taken to reach each milestone are progress too. These smaller, often daily achievements are where the *real* wins lie. They should be celebrated too.

*

It's easy to take your daily progress for granted. Sometimes it's so slow, you can't even see it. Not until all those days add up to a year and you realise you've gone from walking round the block to running five kilometres.

I like to call life progress 'life wins'. For me, they can be as big as landing a magazine cover, or as simple as getting everyone showered and down for bed for the night, getting through a hard day, making it to a gym class, taking a call with a friend. A life win is an attitude – doing something that makes you feel good about yourself – not how big or small the task is.

Whatever your goal, celebrating small wins along the way is key to success. It motivates you to keep showing up. For example, when I'm in the gym and manage to increase my weights, I feel proud of my small accomplishment. I take a moment to acknowledge and celebrate it. Even though it might not seem like much, I know it's leading to a far bigger goal – I'm getting stronger and better. Every small improvement leads to gains.

Getting the kids to school is progress. Ultimately it should result in the big goal: getting them an education. But along the way there are so many small, beautiful goals – the reasons to show up every single day. The first time they read you a book. Make a new friend. Share their news in front of the class. Make the sports team, the school play, finish their homework, eat all their lunch, take the teacher flowers. It's so much more than school. All the while, they're learning how to be in the world. And you? You're learning patience and how to be the love. Celebrate that. It's worth it.

I love hosting people at my house. I'm always having my sisters, nieces and nephews over and I absolutely adore it. My family comes over almost every weekend. The music's on and we catch up, play games, eat food and just hang out. It's our weekly catch-up to celebrate the consistent hard work we've each put in.

Sometimes, wins can be the smallest of things. I've always been a terrible sleeper, so getting a good night's sleep is progress. Every time I sleep well, I know I'm helping my mental health and repairing muscle. At first, I couldn't even count on sleep. My first steps were the tiniest of wins, really just adjustments to my sleep routine: no screentime, taking a bath, going to bed at the same time, meditating instead of panicking that I'm still awake. By making these small changes, my sleep gradually improved. Little, by little, by little.

Once you start noticing life wins, you'll never stop celebrating them. Good hair day? Win! Early to a meeting? Win! A parking space near the front door? Win! Dropping your phone and it doesn't crack? Amazing!

I've heard that people are always waiting to get good news. Waiting. Waiting. Still waiting . . . What are they waiting for?

300

There's good news coming our way *all the time*. It's in all the little things. So don't let the life wins pass you by.

Counting life wins

Thinking back over the past day or two, list your small wins – as many as you can!

....

....

....

....

....

....

....

....

Let's get this
party started.

THE BIG WINS

Small life wins are a delightful, constant drip-feed of positivity into your day. And they're great! But sometimes, you just can't beat the *big* ones. Whether to rejoice in a huge achievement, or simply celebrate a personal milestone, there's *always* a good reason to celebrate *large*. Besides, who doesn't love a party?

*

I am incredibly fortunate that I've had so many reasons to celebrate. Once past their teething problems, Tammy Fit and Saski went from strength to strength. Then came endorsements, major magazine covers, interviews and being flown around the world for appearances and events. Wave after wave of exciting milestones continue; most recently, the birth of my third beautiful baby, Posy. Ten weeks after she was born, we featured on the cover of *Forbes* magazine. There's been a *lot* to cheer.

It's hard to believe that when I first started out it was just me sitting at home with my PDFs and my laptop. The early years juggling fledgling businesses and tiny babies were super tough. Breaking up with the kids' fathers brought a whole new set of challenges, and I've said as much as I'm ever going to say about *that* party. But among the highs and lows, I've always made it a point to celebrate. Even when I've been down, I've had love and support. I could see the progress I was making on my journey.

Personal milestones like birthdays, weddings, anniversaries, babies and graduations end up being the biggest celebrations because they involve both the *heart* and the *journey*. Thirty years is a good time to reflect back on and celebrate all the amazing things one has achieved to get to that point – all the wins, experiences and progress. Never hesitate to throw a party to celebrate big occasions. They are, seriously, the best.

At those times, take a moment to stand back and soak it in. When I look around at my family and loved ones having fun and being together, I'm overcome with gratitude. It makes me realise just how blessed I am. More than a photo, pausing to allow that full-body emotion to wash through you will stay with you for a long, long time after the party is over. So take a minute, it'll last a lifetime.

The big celebrations
Write out a time you celebrated big! Enjoy remembering every detail.

....

....

....

....

....

....

Happy holidays everyone! ♥ 🎄✨ These times are so, so precious so don't forget to dance, sing, love & hold the ones you love close. Sending some extra love to anyone needing it this time of year. 🫶🫶

Make time to
not know or care
what day it is.

HOLIDAYS

I love celebrating by buying gifts for others. I don't mind getting them myself, either! But more than *objects*, I love *experiences*. And holidays may be my favourite experiences of all.

Physically removing yourself from work and switching off the phone transports you to another place. Everything becomes centred on enjoyment – for you, your family and your travel mates. All day, all night happiness. What better way to celebrate life? In this state of bliss, you program only good things into your mind, body and soul. No wonder we feel amazing after going away. Making time to *not* know or care what day it is, is just as important as chasing your goals.

*

When work and life become crazy-busy, planning a holiday with my family is the perfect antidote. Knowing that you have an escape hatch ahead is motivation gold. Whether we're talking a big trip overseas or a weekend staycation – they *all* count. Each one is worth it.

Holidays miraculously slow . . . everything . . . down. They remind us to enjoy life rather than continuously try to 'make it happen'. Life unfolds of its own accord, whether we think we're in control or not. Holidays help us let go of chasing dead-lines and appointments and allow life to flow and do its thing. It's amazing how when you let go of the reins, the world keeps showing up.

When we lived in Singapore with Mum and my step-dad Nathan we travelled a lot because it was so easy to get to places. Travel is such an incredible teacher because you get to fully immerse yourself in another culture and do things you wouldn't normally do. Once we stayed in a haunted castle in Bath, England with about thirty family members. It was such an incredible, hilarious time and I'll treasure those memories forever.

These days, I love taking my kids on big family holidays. And I have to say they've got a lot better at travelling! As babies, they would cry for five hours straight on the plane. Now they're good, as long as they're occupied. Just make sure you bring the travel essentials: a portable charger, face mask, moisturiser, eye cream and water for me; snacks and activities for the kids. A change of clothes is helpful – someone will usually spill some-thing. When we arrive at our destination, I'll have planned some activities and sightseeing, but I like to leave our calendar fairly open to let spontaneity work her magic.

There's a great quote, 'Once a year, go someplace you've never been before.' I love that. See the world as much as possible. But also, go back to places you love. There's some-thing wonderful about getting to know another part of the world *properly*.

The best way to celebrate the moment is to be *in* the moment. Combining that with a fun day in a beautiful setting with the people you love most? That's the *best* kind of celebration.

Missing my babies so unbelievably much, so so so excited to get home and squeeze them. But overall, first child-free vacay in years was a success! 🧖‍♀️ It's honestly been unforgettable. Ya girl is recharged!! ☀️☀️☀️

Just. Book. It.

Wherever, whenever, whatever. Find a destination you've dreamt of and make an actionable plan to get there. Figure out a savings plan, book time off work, learn the language – whatever you need to do. If you can dream it, you can go.

I want to go to: ....

....

With: ....

....

Because: ....

....

And I can't wait to: ....

....

So I am booking it for this date: ....

....

Okay, a little
glitz and glam
is fun.

LIVING (AND DRESSING) IT UP

I like to feel strong, but I'm also incredibly girly. I absolutely love to get dressed up and live it up on occasion. For the right occasion. Knowing what to wear in every circumstance means finding your own personal style then adjusting it to suit the mood of the event. What looks good on you may look terrible on me and vice versa. So have some fun figuring out what looks you love!

*

I've always loved fashion. My sister Emilee led the way in our family. She started her first label quite young and made it her own, and I love her style. She is one of the main reasons I was inspired to start Saski. Even now, every time we start planning a new line I get super excited and can't wait to launch. Clothes are so much fun and I love playing with fashion.

I wasn't always that way. Back when I was finishing high school I was a total hippy and never wore shoes. I liked tie-dyed, loose clothes and floating around like a total beachy chick. After I got pregnant with Wolf, I started dressing up and wearing heels. I guess it made me feel a bit more glam. It was a reinvention, for sure, as I continued developing my signature style.

313

After that I got a *lot* more girly, dressing up in skirts and actual dresses, wearing more make-up and keeping the heels. Nowadays, I would say my style is a mix of both – casual and maybe a little bohemian *and* glamorous and super girly. Plus activewear and swimwear looks, naturally.

I have my staples: jeans, a white crop, leggings and sports bra (so easy, and you can make it look cute with accessories or a handbag), denim jacket, white sneakers (go with everything!) and one classic handbag. Those basics can get me through most days feeling confident and very 'me', but the special outfit for the special occasion is something else altogether.

In my line of work, I attend some amazing events, in amazing places, with amazing people. The hard part is deciding what to wear. Getting ready takes time too, but once you're there, it's always fun. The fashion, fitness and entertainment industries definitely know how to put on a spectacle. For a red carpet, I will dress for the occasion and give it a Tammy twist. I love accessories and make-up, so even if my outfit is quite simple – a sexy dress and heels – I make it my own. Sometimes I like a long, hugging silhouette, at other times, short but classy. Add a designer bag and jewellery and I'm good to go.

There are so many places and ways to celebrate and dressing up is all part of the fun.

Your signature look

Before you can lock in your personal style, it pays to clear out the mess. Follow these steps for a brand new you.

1. Cull your wardrobe. (Yes, you can do it. Including that t-shirt from the girls' weekend in Bali with the cocktail stain.)

2. Keep what you love and give the rest to charity.

3. Make a list of your current staples.

4. Book that night out . . .

Have a good
belly laugh
at least once
a day.

FUN

Is it just me, or do you sometimes feel compelled to do something or say something funny to relax an over-serious crowd? When did we all turn into stiff-suited robots? Kids aren't like that. They understand fun. *Everything* is about fun for them – another reason I love motherhood.

Kids know that poo and fart jokes *are* funny. Also, impersonating pirates, throwing peas across the table, water fights and making Santa beards from bath bubbles.

Kids are smart like that. Studies show that children laugh a lot more than adults which is no surprise to me. They see life in simpler terms. Yet once upon a time we were just like them. Back in the day, we thought a puddle and a stick were the most entertaining things in the world. They still are! Smooshing mud all over your sister's face is hilarious!

Finger painting is fun. So is going on the swings, bouncing on a jumping castle, water slides and pulling the stupidest faces you can to make each other laugh. Acting like a kid isn't immature, it's wise. So don't take yourself too seriously and have some fun!

*

If you're lucky enough to be a parent, you'll have the opportunity to laugh and play with your kids all the time. And guess who's in charge – you! So you can stop whatever else you're doing and join in the fun! And when they're at school? No need to get boring then. Of course we have responsibilities, but if you're not having a great week I can almost guarantee what's missing. Fun.

Beyond champagne with the girls and romantic getaways, fun is usually right at your fingertips. We have tons of fun in our office and I love it that way. At lot of my staff are friends from school days, and we still act as silly as we used to at lunchtime. We play games in the office, make funny TikToks, tell our worst jokes. Everyone deserves to have an upbeat, great day as often as possible.

Individually, it's important to give yourself those fun breaks too. Ring a friend who makes you giggle, watch a comedian for ten minutes, flick through your phone memories and reflect on a great night out when you laughed until you cried.

I read once that you should have at least one good belly laugh a day. Think of it like a dose of medicine, which it is, chemically speaking. Doctors recommend we regularly have a good giggle to relieve tension and stress as it releases happy neurochemicals. Generate those happy chemicals as often as you can because fun is a wonderful, free and easily accessible celebration.

Fun times ahead

What really makes you laugh, gives you joy and is fun?

	Weekdays	Weekends
With kids		
At work		
Friends/family		
By myself		

Reward
yourself - all
the time.

EVERYONE
<3 REWARDS

We're taught from a young age that *motivation* + *effort* equals *achievement* + *reward*. Nice – when it happens. Reality is, life doesn't always work out that way. It's filled with circumstances, relationships, agendas and egos that have nothing to do with you and which you have little control over. So when external rewards come to you – great! Lap them up and be grateful for them. But don't sit around waiting for someone else's praise. The most reliable reward and recognition is *internal*. You can always count on you.

*

As a child, you may have been rewarded for picking up your toys, or getting good grades, or looking after your sister. These are all *conditional*. You may equally have had privileges withheld or even been punished for 'bad' behaviour. Also conditional.

If you thought that was tough, try being an adult. Even when you have justly earned your reward, it may never come. Wage increases are few and far between when the economy is tight, no matter how hard you work. While money can help materially and is *always welcome* in my book, because it's tied to societal factors, our ability to influence it can be limited. Not impossible,

The balance between having a thriving career & spending time with my kids.

The balance between having a wholesome home life & a vibrant social life.

The balance between pushing myself & stopping to embrace how far I've come.

The balance between doing what I love & making money.

The balance between working all night & taking time to rest.

The balance between being independent & asking for help.

Whatever it is, make sure you find YOUR balance.

since beliefs and action play a big part, but not guaranteed – at least, not to arrive exactly when and how you need it. Relying solely on such external rewards can be disheartening.

Rewarding yourself in other ways is essential to maintaining motivation. It's why I'm so keen on celebrating all wins – big and small. Achieving a goal is its own reward. The feelings that success generates – relief, freedom, elation – can be unmatchable. Does anyone ever forget the exhilaration of finishing their last-ever school exam? Walking out of those gates one final time to begin the rest of their life? Complete and utter joy!

Landing that deal, signing that contract, watching your sales climb and climb and climb is such a wonderful feeling. The income is welcome, but knowing all the hard work and effort you've put into making that happen is a huge part of the payoff. When you catch yourself standing in a real-life moment you have visualised for so long, savour it: crossing that finish line, cradling your newborn, hosting your first dinner party. Each one should be cherished and celebrated! It's these moments that make life so sweet.

Years ago I read that setting small, achievable goals towards the big goal was key to success. Not just setting them, but taking a moment to reward each one as you reached it. I do that now on a daily basis. For example, once the kids are dropped off, I reward myself with a peaceful moment of breathing deeply and centring myself. When I finish my workout, it's a yummy meal. Dressing each day, I choose an outfit I love as the reward. A cup of coffee after that big meeting? Reward! You may already be having many similar moments across your day, but are you acknowledging them with rewards? It's amazing how powerful reframing them can be. An appreciation (aka gratitude) mindset offers proven benefits that can help improve sleep, mood and immunity. So reward yourself and bask in the halo effect.

I'm a huge fan of meditation. I love travelling, but real life doesn't always allow it. When I'm desperate for a break, but can't get away, I take ten minutes to imagine myself somewhere far away. My favourite location is a white sandy beach with turquoise water. I close my eyes, breathe deeply and immerse myself in the scene. Using all my senses I imagine the smell of the sea, the feel of the breeze, the taste of fresh juice, the sound of the waves, the colour of the water. In no time at all, my heart rate has dropped, my mind has cleared and I'm ready for the next challenge.

All rewards matter, mostly because they make you feel good about yourself. It's a way to celebrate you, every day. Every single thing you achieve, every positive piece of energy you give, every little step of progress in your life.

Reward yourself

Think about your average day: in what ways can you start giving yourself rewards? It could be that you already are, you're just not thinking of them in that way, or that you need to include more.

Morning reward: ....

Mid-morning reward: ....

Midday reward: ....

Afternoon reward: ....

Evening reward: ....

After-dinner reward: ....

Live a grateful
life.

GRATITUDE

While it's made a few appearances throughout this book, as we reach a close, I think gratitude deserves its very own chapter. To me, it's the perfect way to end. Of all the ways to celebrate life, gratitude is the best.

Gratitude is a warming internal hearth you can visit whenever you need. No matter what you're going through, if you can find something to be thankful for, gratitude will soften your mood. Gratitude makes everything good and worthwhile. It gets me up in the morning, it gets me through hard parts of my day and it's the last thing I think about each night. It reminds me that the glass is half-full.

Gratitude helps you see the whole point. If you take one thing away from *Show Up*, I hope it's this: practise gratitude. Every day. Make it a habit to appreciate yourself and everything and your view on life will change.

*

It's so easy to feel gratitude. All you have to do is reflect on all you've been through. What you've survived, what you've learnt, what you've achieved, who's loved you and whom you've loved. Everything that's made you the person you are today.

Sitting here today in my home in southern Queensland, I'm thinking about that rainforest valley not far away, the place where I grew up. I'm so grateful for my wild and creative upbringing, for my dad and sisters and everything we shared. We didn't have luxuries, but we had music and laughter, our imaginations, and buckets of love. To me, that was everything. That life taught me to be grateful for what I have.

I'm thinking about Singapore and all those places we went overseas and the huge, incredible learning curve of living with Nathan and Mum and all my siblings. International school. What a mind-blowing experience that was! My step-dad's library and everything I learnt there. I am so incredibly grateful for all of that. I think both lifestyles – nature child and international jetsetter – made me see life from many angles and appreciate all of them.

Then there's the hard times at uni, the break-ups and my LA chapter. All that challenge and heartbreak. It may sound funny, but I am so incredibly grateful for those experiences too. I think the toughest times reveal your real character – make you who you are. They taught me so much, but most of all, they taught me even *more* gratitude for what I have, and to be strong.

I am grateful that I picked myself up all those years ago, nineteen years old and pregnant, with little more than an idea, a small library's worth of knowledge, and a lot of determination. I'm grateful that girl had her heart broken a few times and learnt to pick herself up again. It made her both stronger and softer. And she didn't do it alone.

Which brings me to my deepest gratitude, because it isn't about the career or the achievements or the stuff you've got or even the things you overcame, it's the people who helped you get here. The people you love and who love you.

I'm so, so grateful to my sisters . . . I get teary even trying to write the words because where would I even be without them? *Who* would I be without them? I don't even know. Then there's

Your effort to continuously improve should never stop. Whether that is through trying to be a kinder person, exercising more, reading a new book, showing more gratitude. Be grateful for every day, for the chance to live, for every human emotion and experience. While remembering that nobody is perfect and that there is always room for growth.

my mum and my dad and my brothers. My kids. My heart is so, so full when I think about them.

I have a beautiful life, glittering and fulfilling, yet all of that, *all of it*, would mean nothing without their love. It is what has got me here and what has gotten me through. Gratitude is the sweetest thing. Gratitude for the past and gratitude for the present and gratitude for the future too, because there will be more adventures ahead, more mistakes and heartbreak, more triumph, laughter and total joy.

What are you most grateful for?

As my last tip for you, I wanted this one to be super special. This is something I do at the end of every single day: a gratitude daydream. Before I go to sleep, I go through all the things I am grateful for. It's funny how that changes each day because other nice thoughts float in and out, yet – they are always about the people I love. I hope you adopt the habit too because the more you practise gratitude, the better you'll get at it. And the more beautiful your life will be.

Q & A

I get asked a lot about my life – some kind questions, some critical, some curious and some a bit out there. I've tried to address the big questions throughout this book, but here are a few extra. Snuggle into your comfy couch because it's time for Q & A!

If you had your time over, would you still do the whole influencer thing?

This is such a good question and it really made me think. But yes. If I had my time over I would *definitely* do the whole influencer thing again. It was the perfect opportunity for me – it suited who I was, where I was, and it worked out brilliantly. I've been incredibly lucky and I'm very grateful for it.

Despite the trolls, sharing aspects of my life along the way with Instagram and YouTube has also been really fun. It's amazing to see my life unfold in snippets and pictures and reels, like a mini-documentary. Whenever I need a pick-me-up I scroll through my feed and smile. It's impossible not to be cheered by that. Honestly, I feel very fortunate.

Do you compare yourself to other influencers and feel the need to compete?

It's funny how some people seem to think that there's this secret society of influencers and we're all in competition with each other. Spoiler alert: there isn't and we aren't! I do enjoy following some people, but most of my time is taken up just trying to be me, delivering positive motivation and fashion inspiration, and taking care of my family. I don't really have time to spend worrying about what other people are up to.

It comes back to that saying, 'Comparison is the thief of joy'. There will always be someone out there doing something amazing. It might become the next big thing in my sphere and that's fine. But I always say, it's better to focus on yourself. It's easy to look at what others are doing and compare your own career to theirs, but that will get you absolutely *nowhere* except perhaps to a place of envy or insecurity.

You can be inspired by other people, but at the end of the day no-one is you and no-one is bringing what you bring to the table. You're unique and so are they. *There's room for everyone.* Being jealous and petty seems pretty ridiculous to me. Use your energy to work on yourself and your goals rather than worrying if someone else's grass is greener. The only person you should compare yourself to is the person you were yesterday.

How do you handle being criticised about getting your body back in shape so quickly after having your babies?

This media story has been a particularly painful part of my journey and my motivations for getting my body back in shape, and my actual physical ability to do so, have been completely misunderstood by some people.

To start with, I have *always* worked out both before and during my pregnancies, so my body was always going to be in a good position. I didn't have a huge amount of choice – I needed to do it at some point as that's what my businesses are built on:

my health and fitness routines and my fashion line. But that's *my choice for me*, not anyone else. I don't think all women should try to do what I did because not all women spend the majority of their mornings in the gym.

Posting a before-and-after story about my own journey ten months after Po was born, then waking up to headlines screaming that I was promoting 'unrealistic standards', was the last thing I expected or wanted. My postpartum routine has been realistic for me because I'm used to training like that and my body is used to it too. I never expected or wanted other mums to feel that kind of pressure. Everybody is different and every one of us has different lives, opportunities and priorities.

Those were my goals. I am used to feeling strong and I love it. I am fortunate that my body has muscle memory after all these years and responds quickly. I'm also in the habit of eating and training the way I do, so the post-baby workouts were just part of normal life for me.

The absolute *last thing* I want is for any mum out there to feel pressured into getting their body back to where it was quickly, if at all. My situation is pretty unique. All I wanted to do was offer advice, help and motivation for people, wherever they were at. Hopefully I achieved that and I'm very sorry if I made anyone feel bad in any way. My intention was genuinely the opposite.

Staying active during my pregnancy definitely helped A LOT when it came to rebuilding my strength after Po. One thing to note: I am not saying you should aim to look like this, this is my personal journey. Feeling strong is the goal here. 👋 💪

Q & A

Who inspires *you?*
Plenty of people have inspired me in my life, and for different reasons, but I would like to especially mention my sister Amy. She really inspires me. She's incredibly hard-working and that's something that has always impressed and motivated me. She's also really generous and has helped me so much I swear, I seriously don't know what my life would have looked like without her.

Does it ever get to a point where you feel your influence is getting too big?
Sometimes the weight of being followed by millions of people does feel a bit heavy. Sure, I know that being an influencer means you *do have influence*, but it's a very big responsibility when there's literally millions of people reading what you say and observing what you do. However, at some point you need to do your job, go out on a limb and put yourself out there. That's the nature of the game I'm in and you can't overthink it too much or you'll go insane!

I will say this though: there's a dark side to social media. The images of perfection are endless, which is why I take on board the feelings of new mums feeling insecure and judged by my own post-baby fitness regains. What you see on social media is only one person's journey and you can't compare yourself to that in any real sense.

It's only what people are willing to show you, after all, which is completely self-censored. Smoke and mirrors, as they say. It's one of the reasons I try to keep it real, by making sure I post moments of struggle in my own life as well – the not-so-pretty side of things. It's part of the influence I want to have: emphasising that neither me nor my life are perfect *at all*.

This may also sound funny coming from an influencer, but sometimes I think you really need to take a break from social media, especially if it's starting to impact you negatively. If you're being saturated with imagery and messages that make you feel inadequate or bad about yourself, you need to shut it down, or rebalance it with plenty of other positive messaging.

If you *do* choose to do a lot of social media, remember that we influencers are just that: online influences. It's up to you to choose what to take on board, or not. Ultimately? Trust in yourself. That's the influence that will always count the most.

I'm at the point in my life where I feel like nothing could shake me and that gives me such a feeling of PEACE.♡ It's been a long road to get to this and of course I still have down days or moments where it can all get a bit overwhelming. From non-stop work to running around after 3 kids and everything in between. But training, practising gratitude daily, prayer, allowing time for reflection and cup-fillers, and even the painful moments – it's all led me here. To feeling probably the best I have felt in years. It's been such a long road, yet somehow it's still the beginning. 🫶

EPILOGUE

There will never be a point where I wake up and say, 'Okay, that's me done, I'm *exactly* where I want to be.' Not financially, not spiritually, not mentally. As long as I'm alive, I resolve to be better than I was yesterday and become the best version of myself. To me, that is hugely motivating.

Right now, however, I'm just happy to stand and look out the window and feel gratitude, because I've realised I'm at one of those rare crossroads in life. I don't think there's anything that could throw me right now. I feel strong, *really* strong, and it's because of all that love in my life.

It's bittersweet to watch my babies getting older, but I'm looking forward to seeing them grow and continuing to grow alongside them. I'm looking forward to purchasing or building my forever home in the coming years and travelling to places I've never been. I'm looking forward to expanding my businesses and have high hopes about the direction they're going in. Right now, life is exciting and it will be exciting in the future. Meanwhile, every single day is packed full of amazing moments. Every day has something to offer and look forward to.

I feel like it's taken me many years to get to the point I'm at now, and yet I'm only just approaching thirty. It's been a big life already and anything can happen, but I'm not afraid because I have all that love around me, keeping me strong.

My advice to you, as you close the pages of this book, is to remember all the lessons *you've* learnt during your own journey so far. You have built the person you are through every decision, every emotion and every experience you've ever had. Keep backing and believing in that incredible being, okay? And don't ever let yourself take no for an answer. If you do those things, you'll find your big dreams are right within your reach.

Most of all? Live a grateful life. It's worth showing up for that.

ACKNOWLEDGEMENTS

Firstly, I want to say thank you to my wonderful family. To my mum Nathalie and my dad Mark, for bringing me into this world. Without you both I would not be the person I am today. I love and appreciate you so much and I hope I am making you proud. And to my step-dad Nathan, for showing me that success isn't something out of my reach.

To my sisters and brothers, Amy, Emilee, Starlette, Henri, Ava and Maximus – thank you for always being my safe place. For always being by my side and showing up for me when I need you. There are no words to describe how much you all mean to me. Also to Amy, as my business partner – I appreciate you so much and wouldn't be where I am without you. Thank you for inspiring me every day with your hard work, love and wisdom.

To my children, Wolf, Saskia and Posy – you are my heart outside of my body. You have taught and continue to teach me every day what it means to be human. You have taught me about myself, about life, about love and about what truly matters in this world. I love and cherish you endlessly and I'm so grateful I get to be your mama.

To my fiancé Matthew, thank you for bringing so much love and laughter into my life and for being such a kind, loving partner.

You're one of the best people I've ever met and I love you more than you know.

To my Tammy Fit and Saski teams – thank you for being you! The fact that I get to have so much fun at what I call work is all because of you. Your passion and effort is never unnoticed.

I also want to say a huge thank you to my amazing community/fans/followers. Without you none of this would be possible. I pinch myself every day when I think how lucky I am to be able to connect with so many amazing people all over the world. I am so very grateful to you all for coming along on this journey with me and giving me so much purpose.

And lastly, to Penguin Random House and your amazing team, for bringing something I have wanted to do for so long to life. Thank you for making this dream come true.